THE SAG

The
Saga Health Guide
Dr J.A. Muir Gray

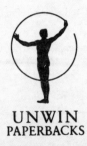

UNWIN
PAPERBACKS

LONDON SYDNEY WELLINGTON

First published in Great Britain by Unwin Paperbacks,
an imprint of Unwin Hyman Limited, 1988.

Unwin Hyman Limited
15–17 Broadwick Street, London W1V 1FP

Allen & Unwin (Australia) Pty Ltd
8 Napier Street, North Sydney, NSW 2060, Australia

Allen & Unwin New Zealand Pty Ltd with the Port Nicholson Press
60 Cambridge Terrace, Wellington, New Zealand

British Library Cataloguing in Publication Data

Gray, Muir
  Saga health guide. – (Saga Guides)
1. Old persons health self care
I. Title   II. Series
613'0438
ISBN 004 440170 1

Set in 12 on 13 point Plantin by Columns, Caversham, Reading
and printed in Great Britain by Cox & Wyman Ltd, Reading

CONTENTS

THE SAGA HEALTH GUIDE

1 GOING FOR HEALTH AFTER RETIREMENT

This book has been written to help you to better health. It focuses on the opportunities for improving health before and after retirement and is based on one simple principle – namely, that most people can improve their health no matter how old they are. There are several factors influencing health which look very simple in the introduction to a book such as this, but which may be more difficult to achieve in practice. These factors (which are, in fact, as relevant for people in their twenties or thirties) are:

1 Good housing and good income – these are foundation stones for good health.
2 The way you live influences your health and a healthy lifestyle can improve your health.
3 Hidden health problems need to be found and dealt with.
4 Health and Social Services are there to help you to better health.
5 Even if you develop a disease you can respond healthily to that disease by coping with it and not letting it beat you.
6 Keeping active and involved with other people enables you to develop as an individual and this, not merely the absence of disease, leads to good health in retirement.

Because it is not always easy to follow these principles in practice, you may need help and support, and there are many people willing to help you. Usually people think of doctors, health visitors or some other group working for the Health Service as the professionals who can help people to better health, but more important than all these are your family and friends. The importance of families is obvious, but we are only just starting to appreciate how much retired people can do to help one another. They can do this in a number of different ways.

For example, a group of retired people may change their lifestyle in some way that leads to better health – perhaps by deciding to go away together, to try something new: pony trekking, sailing, swimming or painting. They may discuss ideas of how to get the most out of their income, or they may simply be able to laugh and joke together about the way in which many younger people fail to recognize their worth or their qualities.

Just as other people can help you, so you can help other people. Throughout this book, therefore, I have included pointers to help you help others. Indeed, some of you may already be helping someone close to you who is having a struggle to maintain and improve his or her health. Even if everything in your family is going well, think of what you can do to help others even more than you do at present. Helping other people helps *you* to better health because it challenges your skills and develops your potential.

Ageing – a Normal Process

The objective of this chapter is to help you understand what is happening to your own body as a result

Challenges in old age	Example	Increased effect on older person
Immobility	Being confined to bed by illness	More rapid loss of muscle and bone strength
Dehydration	As a result of diarrhoea and vomiting in food poisoning	Longer recovery time required
Drug treatment	Side effects of drugs used for arthritis	Drug side effects are more common
Infection	Infection in one part of the body, e.g. the bladder	Not only the bladder, but the person's general physical and mental health can be affected.

of the normal process of ageing and to plan what you can do to minimize its effects.

Ageing is a normal biological process which affects all animals. It becomes the dominant biological process when the period of growth and development has come to a stop at the end of adolescence, and should not be thought of as starting at the age of sixty, sixty-five or seventy.

The effects of ageing are many and varied, but the general result is to reduce the body's ability to cope with challenges and changes. For example, the body has a number of mechanisms for responding to alterations in environmental temperature. If the weather turns colder or warmer, your body's internal 'thermostat' turns your 'central heating system' up or down, controlling both the amount of energy you burn and the amount of hot blood passing through the blood vessels of the skin. With ageing, the 'thermostat' works less well, just as is the case with the thermostat in the central heating system in a house. The result of this is that people who are markedly affected by the ageing process may develop hypothermia when the environment is very cold.

You might care to write down some other challenges which affect people more severely the older they are and compare your list with that on page 3.

Does Ageing Cause Disability?

Consider the following cases:

Mrs G. is eighty-three. She goes abroad for her holidays, works independently, helps other people, cycles occasionally, plays bridge regularly and reads a great deal.

Mr S., who is eighty-five, looks after a very large garden with some help with the heavy digging, and spends a considerable amount of time on committees.

Mrs S. is seventy-nine. She is active in local village and church work and does a good deal of baking, some of which is sold for charity. She plays an active part in the organization of the local old people's club.

All these people have been affected by the ageing process for about sixty years, but none of them is significantly disabled. None of them, it is true, is able to do the things he or she could do when they were twenty, but they are independent in the activities of daily living and enjoy a good quality of life. The reason for this is that their bodies are affected mainly by the ageing process which does not cause significant problems until after the age of ninety, and even then not always. They have not been affected by the three other processes which do cause disability and handicap in old age – disease, loss of fitness and social changes such as the drop in income that occurs on retirement.

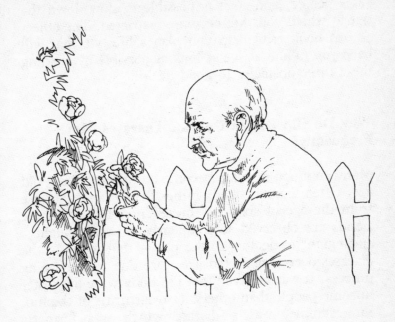

Is There an Elixir of Life?

Before discussing the processes which cause disability, let us consider the ageing process and the claims that have been made that the process can be slowed down.

Since the beginning of time, human beings have searched for an elixir of life, a substance which would slow the ageing process and give eternal life. Even today some people claim to have discovered how ageing can be slowed, usually by following some special diet. There is, however, no evidence that diet or anything else can delay ageing, a fact that will probably come as a relief to most readers. Yet much can be done to influence the rate at which fitness is lost, to reduce the chances that disease will strike and to prevent the social changes that adversely affect older people, and so it is possible to slow down the rate at which your life becomes restricted. The object of this book is to help you plan a lifestyle that will keep you fit and active as long as possible by tackling these three obstacles to good health.

Why Do Old People Develop Diseases More Frequently?

Many common diseases become more common in old age. Often this is a steady rather than a rapid increase from the age of sixty-five or seventy. Because these trends are observed so frequently, it was thought – and taught to doctors in the past – that many of the diseases occurring in old age were due to the ageing process. It was believed that the body wore out faster in some people than others. Osteoarthritis of the hip, for example, was a disease which was formerly thought to be due to a form of accelerated ageing, but it should have been obvious to the medical profession that this idea was false. There was, in fact, a joke in a nineteenth-century edition of *Punch* which should have alerted doctors to the fact that osteoarthritis, and many other diseases, were not primarily due to the ageing process. The caption of this joke ran as follows:

Old woman: Doctor I have a terrible pain in my right knee.
Doctor: It's your age I expect, Mrs Mactavish.
Old woman: Well, my left knee is the same age and it isn't painful, Doctor.

We now know that arthritis is due not simply to the fact that ageing takes place faster in some people than others but to other factors which often affected the person at a young age – for example, a poorly set leg fracture can lead to arthritis in the hip on the same side in later life by placing unnatural strains upon the joint.

Another disease that becomes more common as we age is cancer, and it was once thought that cancer was in some way related to the ageing process, perhaps because the ageing body was less able to detect and knock out cancers at an early stage in their development. It is now known that this is untrue and that the reason why people get cancer more frequently the longer they live is simply that they are around longer and therefore have been exposed for a longer period of time to factors which cause cancer. Most cancers are caused by factors in the environment, or in our diet, or by cigarette smoking; the person who has been smoking for forty years, for instance, is obviously more likely to develop cancer than the person who has only been smoking ten years, or not at all.

Changing Patterns of Disease

As the environment changes so do the diseases that are seen in old age. Men started cigarette smoking in large numbers following the First World War and this social trend was followed by a disease trend as men developed lung cancer, heart disease and the other diseases related to smoking. Many of the disabilities among people who are very old today are the result of cigarette smoking and this is one of the reasons why women, who smoke less, live longer than men. However, because of the social changes that took place during the Second World War, women started smoking in large numbers after the war and we are now seeing smoking-related diseases, notable lung cancer and heart disease, becoming more common among women. In fact, lung cancer is now decreasing in men and increasing in women, reflecting changes in smoking habits.

Old Age – a Message of Hope

The usual image of old age is of a time of inevitable decline in both physical and mental abilities. The reality is different.

- Ageing is only one of the processes which affect people as they grow older.
- Normal ageing does not severely impair the ability of people to look after themselves until they reach the age of ninety or over.
- The three other processes which cause problems for older people – loss of fitness, social changes and disease are not caused by the ageing process.
- These three causes of disability before the age of ninety can all be positively influenced.
- Even though the best way to prevent disease, loss of fitness and social changes (such as the drop in income that can occur on retirement) is to start early in life, preferably in childhood, there is still considerable scope for promoting health by disease prevention, improving fitness and changing your environment after retirement age.

Thus what is conventionally regarded as old age, the part of life after retirement, is simply a phase of life determined by economists. It is they who decide at which ages men and women should retire, and they do this without any regard to the actual abilities of people in their fifties, sixties or seventies. The retirement age is therefore not a sign that old age is starting, simply a sign that work has finished. Similarly, old age is not a time of irreversible decline but a time when poor health can be improved and good health enjoyed.

2 GOOD FOUNDATIONS

Good housing and a good income are essential foundations for good health. Of course, these factors cannot by themselves guarantee that you will have good health, but if you do not have them life is obviously difficult and good health harder to achieve.

The objectives of this chapter, then, are:

1 To emphasize how important it is to try to improve your housing and maximize your income.
2 To suggest steps you can take to make your housing better for your health.
3 To suggest ways in which you can improve your income.

Housing for Health

The type of housing which can help you to better health:

- Is able to be kept to a temperature of at least 62°F (16°C) within your income.
- Is not a cause of anxiety for you.
- Does not increase your risk of home accidents.
- Does not handicap you by causing problems if you are disabled.

Problems with heating (which is particularly important if you suffer from heart disease or respiratory disease) or difficulties with repairs are the types of problem which commonly cause anxiety and depression. They are usually the result of the fact that your income is too low, but there is often something that can be done to help you in these circumstances.

If you are a council tenant, go to the housing department and ask for help.

If you are a private tenant or an owner-occupier, you will probably find the best source of help and advice at the local environmental health department of your council. Each environmental health department has a housing section and the housing officers are able to give advice on a whole range of problems from difficult landlords to ways in which the house you own can be made safer and warmer. They can also give you information about finding the finance to do the necessary work.

Reducing the Risks of Home Accidents
Home accidents usually occur as a result of a combination of two factors – those relating to the individual and those relating to the environment.

Home accidents happen more often to people who are frail. If you are strong, fit and healthy, you are much less likely to suffer an accident at home than if you are weak and frail, so all the advice about good health in this book is relevant to the prevention of home accidents. Perhaps the most important chapter for preventing home accidents is Chapter 4, because the stronger and fitter you are and the better your co-ordination, the less likely are you to trip and fall and the more likely are you to be able to recover your balance if you do happen to lose it.

The risk of accidents also increases if your vision is

poor, but this risk factor can be reduced by taking steps to ensure that you are able to see as sharply as you can (see page 45) and improving the lighting in your house.

Housing and Handicap

If you become disabled, housing that was previously suitable may become unsuitable. For example, a house with an upstairs toilet will no longer be suitable if the occupant becomes unable to climb a flight of stairs. Often is is possible to adapt a dwelling by a simple approach such as putting in a second stair rail, or by much more complex building works such as the installation of a downstairs toilet.

Social Services employ specially trained staff, called domiciliary occupational therapists, who can advise on the best type of alterations in the case of handicap and on the sources of financial help available to fund the work that needs to be done.

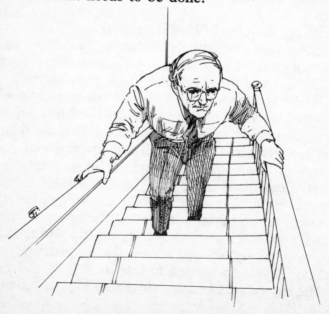

The Saga Property Guide, also in this series, contains many useful tips about ways in which your home can be made warmer, safer and healthier.

Improving Your Income

This book is mainly about good health, but wealth is in general good for your health, and any steps you can take to improve your income or that of people you know can only have a positive effect. If your income is low, you will have difficulty in keeping warm, in buying the foods you need to keep you healthy, and in maintaining your house – and poor housing increases the risk of home accidents. Low income can cause depression and anxiety and, by reducing your opportunities for seeing other people and taking holidays, increase the rate at which you lose fitness, both mental and physical.

If your only income is from social security, ask at the Citizens Advice Bureau or the local Age Concern office to make sure that you are getting all the benefits for which you are eligible. Information on this subject can also be found in *The Saga Rights Guide*. If you have another source of income, for example a part-time job or an occupational pension, ask your bank manager if he or she can suggest any ways you could make your money go further.

Owner-occupiers whose income is inadequate should consider taking out a mortgage to do any work that is needed to improve their home, its heating or its safety, or to carry out repairs which are the cause of anxiety or worry. If you have no family and no one to leave your house to, you should discuss with your bank manager the various schemes that are available to help owner-occupiers make good use of their capital by obtaining an annuity. Even if you have someone to whom you want to leave money, investigate ways in which even part of your capital can be turned into revenue. Often the prospective heir of an older person wants, above all, that older person to spend some money on themselves.

See *The Saga Money Guide*, also in this series, for more detailed information on how you can make the most of your money, and *The Saga Rights Guide* for advice on obtaining all the benefits to which you are entitled.

3 HEALTHY LIFESTYLE

The health of an individual is a product of the many different factors which are listed on page 1. One of these is your lifestyle, which is created by the choices you make about how you will live. Wherever you live, whatever your income, there are certain choices open to you. For some people it is easier to choose one option rather than another, but everyone faces the same choices and this chapter examines these choices and considers the evidence for one being healthier than another.

The objectives of this and the following two chapters are to give information to help you:

1 Consider the choices that can be made in retirement and how these influence health.
2 Make healthier dietary choices.
3 Consider whether to continue smoking or to stop.
4 Choose whether or not to drink alcohol and, if so, how much.
5 Determine how much physical activity you take.
6 Decide how active to keep your mind.

Retirement – the Chance of a Lifetime

Much has been written about the 'problems' of retirement, but what are the true facts?

- Most people enjoy retirement and find that their health improves after they retire.
- The worst thing about retirement for most people is not the loss of the job itself but the drop in income and the loss of friends at work.
- Some of the changes that occur in retirement are the inevitable consequences of stopping work, but many of them result from the decisions that people make about the way in which they wish their life to change.
- The word 'retirement' implies that the person withdraws from life, like a snail drawing into its shell. In fact, this rarely happens. For most people retirement is simply stopping paid employment and for quite a number it means changing from one job to another.

Minimizing the Impact of Retirement

Retirement is a major event in life but, unlike some major events, it can usually be seen coming. If you are aware of the approach of a major change in your life, it is always always helpful to think and talk about this change before it arrives, and the following are useful questions to ask six months before the date on which you are due to retire:

- What will I miss most about work?
- What will be the effect of my drop in income?

Think about these questions and write down the answers, even if they are only a word or two. Then ask five other people whom you know what *they* think you will miss most about work and how you will cope with a reduced income. Don't ask them formally, as if you were doing a survey, but casually during conversation, perhaps over lunch. You may not need to discuss your income with people you do not know well, but you should certainly discuss it with your spouse. As to the first question, 'What will I miss most about work?', some answers you receive may be in agreement with your own, but almost certainly other people will have a different view of how you might react and this will help you in thinking and talking about your retirement.

If you are offered the opportunity at work to go on a pre-retirement course or join a group, take it; although it must be said that some of these courses and groups consist of fairly boring one-sided talks from 'experts' who do not give the other participants the chance to discuss how retirement might affect them.

Three months before you retire you could give yourself a health check, asking yourself the following questions:

1 What are my main health problems at present?
2 Are there ways in which I could become fitter? (See page 31.)
3 Could my diet be improved? (See page 18.)
4 When did I last have my blood pressure measured? If you last had a normal blood pressure recorded more than five years ago, make an appointment for a blood pressure test (see page 55.)
5 Do I smoke cigarettes? (If the answer is yes, see page 26.)
6 What weight am I? (See page 19.)

For women only:
7 When did I last have a cervical smear test? (See page 52.)
8 When did I last have a mammogram? (See page 53.)

Having reviewed these aspects of your health, you can start to think ahead and plan for retirement. Remember that retirement may be a bigger challenge than you expect, so don't plan to reorganize your life completely as well as retiring. It is useful to write down the things you would like to achieve in the first year after you retire and in the second six months of that year you could include one or two ways in which you could improve your health, such as increasing the amount of exercise you take. It is probably better to leave it to the second six months because you will probably find that the first six months vanish quickly, being taken up with a whole variety of household tasks, travel and the tidying up that inevitably occurs towards the end of one phase in life.

Health Plan for Retirement
Your plan for improving your health in the first year after retirement might include the following:

- Ensuring that your weight does not increase above the level it was on the day of retirement.
- Giving up cigarette smoking.
- Doing more of some form of exercise than you have done for years.
- Trying a new type of hobby that you have never tried before.

Eating More Healthily

One of the aims of this chapter is to help you review your diet and decide if you need to make any changes to improve your health. Many older people quite rightly ask, 'What's wrong with my diet?', arguing that if it had been badly wrong they would never have survived to their present age. This is true: the food most people eat has been satisfactory enough for them to reach old age, but there are still some steps that the majority could take to improve their diet and so improve their health in old age.

For people active and intelligent enough to be reading this book there are only three dietary problems which need to be borne in mind:

- The amount of energy you consume each day, which can affect your weight.
- Your fibre intake.
- Your calcium intake.

What Happens if I Consume Too Much Energy?

Food, which produces the energy the body needs to breathe, move about and work, is fuel – like petrol. If you try to put too much petrol in the car, it overflows because the tank is not elastic; if you try to put too much energy into human beings, the surplus energy is gratefully received and converted into fat. People put on weight when their energy intake is greater than their energy output. They lose weight when their energy output is greater than their energy intake.

AM I OVERWEIGHT?

There are numerous test for obesity but the simplest one is to undress, look in the mirror and be honest.

If you are not overweight, weigh yourself and record your weight and the clothes that you are wearing under the following headings:

Date	Weight	Type of clothing	Shoes on or off

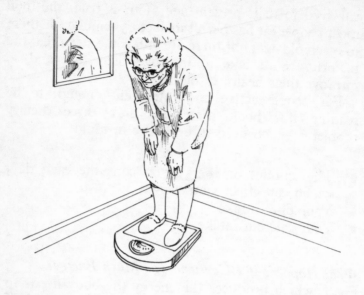

Now set yourself a resolution that you will stay the same weight for the rest of your life. Weigh yourself frequently, always wearing the same type of clothes, about every month or two and record your weight in the same way.

If your weight increases by more than 5 lb (3 kg), or if you notice that it has increased on three consecutive weighings, consider yourself as over-weight and take steps to shed some pounds.

HOW CAN I LOSE WEIGHT?

If you have become aware that you need to lose some weight, you must reduce your energy intake and increase the amount of energy you expend (see Chapter 4). Reducing energy intake will have a quicker effect than increasing energy output, but increasing energy output by adding at least three spells of exercise, each lasting twenty minutes, to your lifestyle each week will make a very important longer-term contribution to weight control.

WHAT ENERGY-RICH FOODS SHOULD BE AVOIDED?
When you eat food, it satisfies two needs. It stops you feeling hungry and it provides the energy your body needs to function. The reason why so many people in developed countries are overweight is that there are many foods now available which contain energy in very small bulk so that it is possible to eat plenty of them without feeling particularly uncomfortable. Three or four hundred years ago you had to eat a tremendous amount of potatoes to consume too much energy for your daily needs. Now that refined carbohydrate (or sugar) is widely available, it is possible to eat a bar of chocolate and consume energy equivalent to that provided by a few pounds of potatoes without the chocolate filling you up in the same way as potatoes did. Therefore it is much easier today to take in too much energy, for which two types of food are especially to blame:

- Those containing sugar (which don't necessarily taste terribly sweet or look sugary).
- Those containing cream and other rich sources of animal fat (which do not necessarily look fatty).

Space does not allow more detailed information here about what foods to avoid to enable healthy weight loss; older people in need of dietary advice or weight control are no different from others and should browse through the wide selection of books available, including *The Saga Food Guide*, also in this series. Knowledge is relatively easy to get; it is the motivation that you put into a diet that makes it work.

WHY SHOULD I LOSE WEIGHT?

Being overweight causes lots of problems in old age, so losing weight now is an insurance for the future. Excess weight increases the risk of accidents, predisposes towards diabetes, aggravates arthritis, reduces your fitness, raises your blood pressure and has a lot of other effects which are better avoided.

SHOULD I TRY A VERY LOW CALORIE DIET?

Very low calorie diets are widely advertised and increasingly popular. They are not likely to cause any harm provided you follow the instructions, but they are not likely to be effective in achieving long-term and permanent reduction in weight. They are useful, although expensive, in helping you to lose a few pounds in weight so that you will look better on the beach on holiday, but they are not the means of achieving a permanent reduction in weight, nor do they suit everyone, so ask your doctor's advice before you embark on a very low calorie diet. Only by changing your diet to healthier foodstuffs rich in fibre and lower in sugar and fat can you do this.

Eating Fibre for Health

It is only in the last hundred years that white flour has become widely available, and it is in roughly the same period of time that we have been able to obtain refined carbohydrate (sugar) from plants which allows us to consume all the energy we need for daily life without consuming as much fibre in grain and vegetables as our ancestors did. For millions of years human beings lived on a diet rich in two types of fibre (cereal fibre and fruit and vegetable fibre), whereas for the past century we have been able to get by while consuming much less of it. Not surprisingly, this has had effects on the body, and it is now recognized that a number of health problems which we see today are due partly or fully to fibre deficiency. Examples include constipation, incontinence and diverticulitis (a condition in which parts of the bowel become inflamed and painful). In addition the risk of developing diabetes is increased, and if a person develops diabetes, fibre deficiency complicates the disease.

DO I EAT ENOUGH FIBRE?
To find out if your diet includes enough fibre, tick the box beside the appropriate answer to each of the following three questions.

1 Do you have wholemeal bread

		Points
All the time?		4
Sometimes but more often than white bread?		3
Sometimes but less often than white bread?		2
Never?		1

2   How often do you eat fresh fruit and/or vegetables with the skin on?

		Points
Daily?		4
Most days in the week?		3
Once or twice a week?		2
Never?		1

3   How often do you have breakfast cereal which contains all the fibre of the cereal?

Every day?		4
Most days of the week?		3
Once or twice a week?		2
Never?		1

Now add up the points for your score. If you have scored over 10 you are probably getting an adequate intake of fibre, although almost everybody would benefit from increasing the amount of fibre they take.

WHAT FOODS ARE RICH IN FIBRE?
Types of food that are rich in fibre are: wholemeal bread; any type of breakfast cereal which states that it contains all the parts of the grain; fruit and vegetables. You can, of course, buy bran which consists solely of fibre and sprinkle this on top of your food, but you should be careful when taking bran because it can have explosive results if you are not used to it and take too much of it.

The Importance of Calcium

The reason why calcium in the diet is so important is that it helps prevent osteoporosis, or bone thinning, in later life which can lead to fractures. People who are more at risk of developing osteoporosis are women, cigarette smokers and those who are very light-boned and petite. Your first preventative step against this condition is to ensure that you are eating plenty of calcium-rich foods.

THE CALCIUM CHECKLIST

Calcium is present in small amounts in many foods, but it is found in large quantities in only a small number of foods, notably dairy foods and tinned fish which has the bones still in it. To discover whether your calcium intake is sufficient, ask yourself the following questions:

1 How much milk do I consume in a week? Award a point for each pint (600 ml) of milk consumed.
2 How often do I have cheese in a week? Give yourself a point for each time you have cheese.
3 How often during a week do I eat tinned fish, such as pilchards, with the bones in? Give yourself a point if you have this food.

Add up these points and if you have more than 10 you are taking in a reasonable amount of calcium. If you are not, you should consider trying to increase your calcium, particularly if you are a woman. There is, however, no easy way of doing this over and above taking a pint (600 ml) of milk a day, because it can be difficult to consume large amounts of foods containing calcium. There are, however, new products available from dairies and the milkman that are rich in calcium and if you can take calcium-reinforced milk several times a week instead of your ordinary milk you will be able to increase your calcium intake dramatically.

There are also two other steps that you can take to reduce your risk of osteoporosis in later life.

If you are a woman, ask your doctor if he or she thinks that you would benefit from hormone replacement therapy after the menopause. Everybody loses bone from about the age of thirty onwards as part of normal ageing, but in women the rate at which bone is lost increases dramatically after the menopause; and those women whose bones are delicate to begin with can have the rate of loss reduced by taking hormones. Hormone replacement therapy carries some risks, and it is therefore important to discuss the balance of risks and benefits with your doctor.

Taking exercise can reduce the rate at which bone is lost. It is well known that bone strength diminishes when people are immobilized in bed – this happens to the young as well as older people – and it does seem that the amount of exercise taken in daily life can determine the rate at which bone is lost. All exercises which require the muscles to be used help the bones stay strong because of the force which the muscles impose on the bones when they contract.

Giving up Smoking

Cigarette smoking is now well recognized as the most common preventable cause of death and disability. What has not been emphasized in the past is the benefit to older people of giving up this habit.

Obviously, if you have been smoking for forty years, your body will have already absorbed a lot of chemicals from cigarette smoke, but it is still the case that, whatever age you are, your health will improve if you stop smoking.

If you give up smoking you will:

- Cope better with cold and influenza.
- Have an easier time with the anaesthetic if you go to hospital for an operation.
- Improve the circulation to your legs; 95% of all amputations of the lower leg are necessitated by cigarette smoking.
- Have fewer symptoms if you suffer from asthma, bronchitis, heart disease, a duodenal or gastric ulcer or intermittent claudication (narrowing of the arteries of the leg).
- Find that your clothes and home will smell more pleasant.
- Save enough money for a good holiday every year.
- Set a good example to your grandchildren and other young people who know you.

One of the best things you can do for your health is to stop smoking.

Will I be Able to Give Up?

Here are a few facts to encourage you to try giving up smoking:

- Most people who give up have tried unsuccessfully to do so before.
- Having tried and failed is not a reason not to try again: some people manage it successfully at the sixth or seventh attempt.
- People are able to give up no matter how many cigarettes they smoke every day: obviously the fewer you smoke, the easier it is, but there are

plenty of records of people giving up after smoking fifty or sixty a day.

- Many people find it easier to give up than they thought it would be.

How Can I Give Up Successfully?

There is no magic formula: everyone finds their own way of giving up smoking, but here are a few tips which you may find helpful:

- Make up your mind that you are going to stop.
- Make an appointment to see your doctor and ask him or her what they think about you giving up; the support of a GP is helpful. The doctor may also be able to give you some leaflets or pamphlets about stopping smoking.
- Set a target date for stopping; tell other people what you plan to do.
- Make a savings plan and collect all the money you would have spent on cigarettes in a box or jar with a definite plan for what you will spend it on.
- See if you can get some people to sponsor you not to smoke and give the money you collect to a charity of your choice.
- When you stop, give up completely – don't try just to cut down. However, if you smoke more than forty a day, you may find it helpful to cut down to twenty a day for two weeks before you stop completely. If you are a very light smoker, you may find it helpful to try to smoke four or five times your usual amount on the three days before you stop smoking.
- Be prepared for the problems that you may face after stopping smoking. Try to avoid smoking at 'danger' times like teabreaks, and for a week or two after giving up, avoid mixing with people who still

smoke and going to places where smoking is common such as pubs. Be very careful after you have had a drink or two as this reduces the commitment to stay stopped.

- Don't sit around doing nothing and feeling tense. Get out and walk or swim or do something with you hands if you feel like a cigarette. Keep things ready for chewing and nibbling such as raw carrots or chewing gum.

- Whatever you do in the first phase after giving up smoking, think of ways in which the amount of exercise you take can be increased. This will not only help you stay stopped, but will also help you deal with any tension you might feel about giving up smoking and help control your weight – a minority of people who stop smoking do experience some increase in weight after stopping.

What About Other Techniques?

Nicotine chewing gum, available on prescription from your doctor, appears to be particularly useful for people who are heavy smokers and who find that they cannot give up by using the approach described in the preceding section. Discuss this option with your doctor if you have tried the method outlined above on a couple of occasions without success.

If you are still having difficulty stopping even after trying nicotine chewing gum, try other techniques such as hypnosis or acupuncture. In the long run everyone stops smoking in his or her own way. What is important is that you keep trying to stop and if you don't succeed once, leave it for six months or a year, summon up your energy and determination and try again, because stopping smoking is the best step you can take to improve your health.

Drinking Sensibly

Alcohol has brought both pleasure and misery to the human race, and has to be used sensibly. As you grow older you may become more sensitive to the effects of alcohol, particularly if you are taking medicines with which alcohol can interact – for example, anti-depressants, tranquillizers or sleeping pills. Hardly anyone who has a drinking problem is aware of it, and one simple measure is to find out how much you drink.

Count a single drink as 1 unit, whether it is a sherry, a glass of wine or half-pint of beer, and add up how many units you have each week. If you drink under 10 units a week, you are drinking in an acceptable range. Between 10 and 20 you need to be careful, and over 20 you should think about reducing your drinking if you want to be healthier.

Sometimes individuals who are depressed or anxious drink more, but do not appreciate that they are doing so. If you see a friend starting to drink heavily, they probably have some sort of problem: do something about it – not by tackling them directly on their drinking, but by saying that you have noticed they are not as happy as they were in the past, and asking if you can help.

4 GETTING OLDER, GETTING FITTER

The word 'fitness' is usually associated with young athletes, but fitness becomes more important the older you are.

What is Fitness?

You are probably sitting down reading this book and it is difficult to judge your fitness when sitting or lying, but if you were to put the book down and walk a mile briskly, or go up and down the stairs five times, you would have to call on your reserves of fitness.

Having fitness is a little like having a bank account. Just as you have money in your pocket or handbag to see you through from day to day, so your body is capable of doing most of the things you want to do on a routine daily basis: getting up, getting dressed, making a cup of tea, walking to the shops, keeping the house tidy and so on. However, when you have to make a big purchase, you have to call on the money in you bank account or building society. Similarly, when you have to do a major piece of work such as climbing four flights of stairs, digging the garden or playing with grandchildren, you have to call on your physical reserves.

People who have plenty of money can buy goods such as a television or a washing machine or have an expensive meal out without too much effort. In the same way people with plenty of fitness can much more easily carry out tasks which require extra strength, stamina, suppleness or skill – the four aspects of fitness – than those who are less fit.

Why Does Fitness Matter?

Fitness matters when you want to do something a little out of the ordinary. If you are at the moment an active person able to walk and cycle or garden, you will need fitness when you are doing extra walking, cycling or gardening.

It is, however, essential to look ahead in life, and if you can build up your fitness now it is just like building up your bank account. You will more easily be able to meet the challenges you may face later on when you reach the age of eighty or ninety.

Look at the health biography diagram opposite. The broken line demonstrates the best possible rate of decline – how somebody like Daley Thompson would decline if he continued to train for eight hours a day.

Now look at the other two lines. Line C represents the decline in ability of Sidney Jones. His interests in life were never very active; he lived in a flat without a garden, always drove to work, and only went for a walk for pleasure once or twice a month and then only round the local park. This lifestyle suited him admirably and he was able to do all that he wanted. Now look at the horizontal line which illustrates the ability level needed to walk a quarter of a mile (0.4 km). Until the age of eighty Sidney was able to do this and thus reached the shops, pub, church and

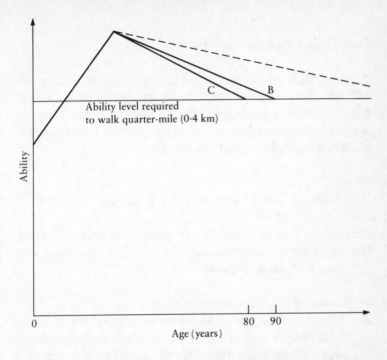

Ability level required
to walk quarter-mile (0·4 km)

Ability

0   80 90

Age (years)

library which were all about a quarter of a mile away from his home. However, there comes a point in his life when he drops below this threshold and is thus cut off from these essentials of everyday life.

Now look at Line B. This represents the decline of Sidney's non-identical twin brother, Jonathan who, without being obsessional about keeping fit, swam once a week, used to cycle down to his allotment at the weekend and who, as a matter of principal, never used a lift unless he had to go up more than three floors. Starting from exactly the same point as Sidney, he declines more slowly and – this is the vital message – he drops below the threshold about ten years later.

The older you are, the more important fitness becomes, and you should start now building up a fitness bank account.

Can Older People Get Fitter?

A great deal of research has been done on fitness in old age, and there is now no doubt that people can be fitter whatever their age. By taking up some type of activity you can change the shape of the line on your health biography and become fitter.

Is it Safe to Try to Improve my Fitness?

People do not develop health problems as a result of trying to get fitter provided that they bear in mind the few rules of safer fitness.

1   Increase exercise levels slowly.
2   Before starting to take more exercise, check with your doctor if you suffer from heart disease, blood pressure or any other chronic health problem.
3   Pick the right kind of exercise.

Some types of exercise are better than others.

- Exercises which involve holding your breath and straining should be avoided; remember that this also includes moving heavy furniture, pushing a car on cold mornings and carrying heavy suitcases. It is better to do exercises which allow you to breathe continuously throughout the period of exercise.
- Exercises which call for very high levels of energy output over short periods of time are better than those which require energy output to be sustained over ten or fifteen minutes rather than over ten or fifteen seconds. High-intensity exercise is parti-

cularly a problem for people who are very competitive because the desire to win may take them past the safety point. Squash is the type of exercise which should be avoided for this reason, unless you are very fit.

- Exercise which involves a lot of banging to the muscles and joints is more likely to lead to problems than exercise which allows muscles and joints to be fully used without banging; for this reason cycling and swimming are better for most people than jogging, and brisk walking is better than running.

How Fit Am I?

There are a number of ways in which fitness can be measured, but the simplest way is to measure it yourself. First, take a watch and measure your pulse rate for one minute while you are sitting down. This is the resting pulse rate. Now you can do a bit of exercise – for example, walking to the shops. Note the time you take to walk from your front door to one of the shops and record which shop is your target. Take you pulse rate when you arrive and note it down when you get back home.

This is not an absolute indicator of your fitness but it would allow you to measure progress. As you become fitter you will be able to walk to the shops either in the same time with less increase in pulse rate, or in a shorter period of time with the same increase in pulse rate, or be able to achieve both – namely, to get to the shops more quickly and with a lower increase in pulse rate.

This test, of course, measures only one aspect of fitness – stamina. It is not meant to measure strength,

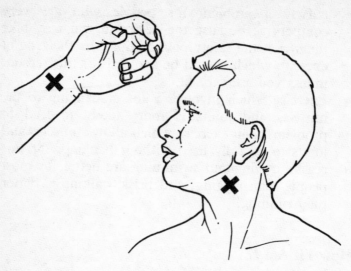

Taking the pulse: X marks the spots where the pulse is most easily felt.

skill or suppleness, which are much more difficult to assess. The best thing is simply to try to improve these other aspects of fitness.

How Can I Improve my Fitness?

There are three ways in which you can get fitter:

1 By taking up some new form of exercise.
2 By choosing fitness activities in your daily life.
3 By carrying out some simple exercises at home.

Choosing an Active Leisure Interest
There is only one rule worth bearing in mind: you must do something that you enjoy.

A wide variety of options is now available for retired people who want to improve their fitness.

Since we are looking at the choices you can make, ask yourself six questions about an activity you are considering taking up:

- Is it safe?
- Will it help improve my strength?
- Will it help improve my stamina?
- Will it help improve my suppleness?
- Will it help improve my skill?
- Will I enjoy it?

Whatever you do, you must be prepared to do something that you find difficult – not painful or uncomfortable, but difficult.

- It is when you feel that little bit breathless, and think you would like to stop but carry on, that you increase your stamina.
- It is when you find what you are doing tiring but carry on that you improve your strength.
- It is when you feel your muscles and joints just start to stretch a little but don't immediately give up that you improve your suppleness.
- It is when you have to try three or four times to perform some new task that you are starting to improve your skills.

Cycling, swimming and dancing are probably three of the most useful types of exercise which many retired people enjoy. However, almost everybody, from professional footballers to older people, tends to choose activities which will improve strength, stamina and skill and ignores the aspect of fitness that is at least as important as these others, namely suppleness.

Why not consider enrolling in a yoga class? It is the best means of improving suppleness. Yoga is not an

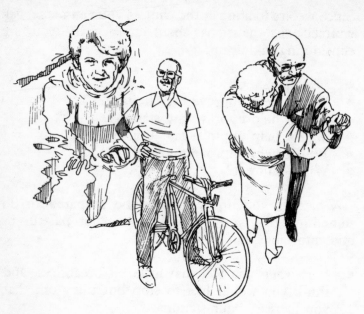

activity reserved for young people. Everybody can benefit from it and it will help you to feel better.

The Fitness Choices
Just remember that in your everyday life you will be offered choices – whether to take the car or walk, whether to use a lift or escalator or the stairs, whether to use a power drill or a hand drill to make a single hole in a piece of wood. At least once a day you should choose the active option.

Your Daily Dozen
Some of you will have exercised every day throughout your life or had parents who did so, and daily exercises are even more important the older you become. Try the following simple exercises twelve times each day. Do them slowly and carefully at first and don't push you joints too far. If you do these

exercises every day to the best of your ability, you will be able to prevent stiffness and maintain suppleness.

SUPPLE SHOULDERS

The shoulder joint can move in almost any direction. Ordinary housework and gardening keep the shoulder supple to a certain extent by in moving it in some directions, but they do not exercise all movements of the shoulder joint, particularly important ones like lifting your hand above your head or reaching your hand round the back of your neck to brush your hair or fasten a necklace.

The simplest and safest way to keep your shoulders as supple as possible is with the following exercise. Slowly swing your arm in a circle, starting with your hand by your side and lifting it slowly forwards and upwards, whilst keeping your elbow straight, until your arm is vertical; at this point it should be brushing your ear. Then, still keeping your elbow straight, move your arm backwards until the circle is complete. Try to do this twenty times every morning with each arm. You may find it difficult at first, but keep going – *carefully*. Do not push your joints into a position you find painful.

Some people suffer a disorder known as frozen shoulder in which there is an inability to lift the arm out sideways or to raise it above the level of the shoulder joint. The type of slow arm-circling exercise described above can help prevent frozen shoulder, and reduce the risk of recurrence if you have had it once. Remember, however, that if your shoulder is painful you should not try to force this movement but should seek your doctor's advice.

KEEPING YOUR KNEES SUPPLE

Once a day lie on the floor, face down, and bend one knee, so that the foot is right up behind the buttock. Repeat this ten times on each leg.

STRETCH YOUR MUSCLES

It is important to stretch your muscles a little every day. One simple way to stretch your leg muscles is to place one leg in front of the other and slightly bend the knee of the leg that is in front, keeping the other leg straight. Now try to raise the toes of the foot that is in front, keeping the heel on the ground, and feel your muscles stretch.

MAKE UP YOUR OWN EXERCISES

You can work out how your muscles and joints move and it is not too difficult to invent exercises with stretch joints. Always remember the following important principles, however:

- Never force a joint.
- Make all your movements slow and steady.
- Stretch your muscles and joints daily.

If you can find the time you should consider taking up yoga, as a good yoga teacher will help you learn how to stretch safely and effectively.

5 KEEPING YOUR MIND LIVELY

Normal ageing does have some effect on the way your mind works, as you will have probably noticed. It becomes more difficult to remember facts, particularly those that you acquired recently: you may forget the name of the man you met yesterday, although you remember the name of your school teacher of sixty years ago. The mind also works more slowly when required to do certain types of tasks.

However, the effects of ageing on the brain have been over-emphasized and if you keep your brain occupied and your mind lively you will not suffer a serious loss of intellectual ability, provided that you are fortunate and do not develop any disease of the brain, such as Alzheimer's. It is very important to remember that Alzheimer's disease, or dementia as it is sometimes called, affects only a minority of old people, and that if you find yourself forgetting names or unable to remember what you went upstairs to fetch, this does not mean that you are developing the disease. If you are worried that you may be developing dementia, you should discuss this with your doctor. But people who are worried that they may be affected very rarely actually are, because one of the early changes during the development of Alzheimer's disease is that the sufferer loses insight and is unable to detect what is going on.

There are two ways in which you can keep your

mind active and lively – stay involved and try learning new skills.

Staying Involved

The best exercise for your mind is 'mind wrestling' – talking, discussing and arguing with other people, and growing old and ageing are not by themselves major problems compared with isolation. Problems develop when the person is able to see and talk with fewer people than they could in times past because of disabling diseases such as arthritis. If you find that you are not going out so often either because of disability or because you are nervous of going out alone at night, try to find alternative ways of staying involved with people – for example, change from an evening to an afternoon bridge club or take up new activities in the afternoon at your local community centre.

Acquiring New Skills

As well as staying involved you should also challenge your mind by acquiring new skills. Older people with grandchildren have this opportunity given to them as their grandchildren may ask them to learn to play Cluedo or chess, or computer games, but is is also possible to find your own source of intellectual stimulation.

One useful approach is to make a new year's resolution every year to learn some new skills. These can involve just your mind, such as learning a new language in preparation for a holiday abroad or joining a group studying a topic such as English; or both mind and body, such as painting, carpentry, weaving or car repairs.

There are many opportunities to obtain new skills and knowledge. You may well receive a leaflet through your door in the early autumn advising you of the classes that are available for adults or you can find out what is available by going to your local community centre or by writing to the adult education advisor at your county education department.

Combining the Two

It is possible both to 'get involved' and acquire new skills by taking up an activity which requires you to work with other people to achieve some change. Many have benefited from the opportunity of retirement to play a more active part in local or national politics by working for their local constituency parties, or by becoming more active in an organization such as the church, a club or voluntary society. Some older people feel that young people rely on them too much to run organizations such as these, but another way to look at this type of work is to consider it as something that will be beneficial to your health as well as helpful to others.

6 BODY MAINTENANCE

Your body is like your car. Your car needs servicing regularly and some people even clean their cars, though that is an optional extra! In the same way that you look after a car you should also develop a programme of caring for your body, and the objective of this chapter is to help you learn about the body maintenance tasks which should be carried out to keep your body in good working order.

These tasks are of two sorts, just like your car maintenance tasks.

First, there are the bits of the body that you can see yourself and care for yourself. Just as you can see the red light come on when your car's oil pressure drops too low and put in oil yourself, you know if your vision is failing and when you need to do something about it. There are, however, parts of your body that can go wrong without your knowing, just as there are parts of your car than can start to fail without its being obvious. The tests that are used to detect these hidden problems are called screening tests and this chapter explains about the screening tests which are useful in old age and how you can get them done.

Keeping Sharp Sight

As a result of normal ageing certain changes take place in the eye. The main one, which affects all people, is that the lens of the eye loses some of its elasticity and cannot adapt so well to change. The result is that many people need two sets of glasses, or bifocals, as they get older. This does not cause significant problems, however, and most people will still be able to read a newspaper in their late eighties or nineties, so long as they take steps to keep their vision as sharp as possible.

Good Lighting, Good Vision

Because the eye becomes less efficient with age, it is necessary to help it by providing a better environment in which it can work. The simplest step to take is to improve lighting either by putting a stronger bulb in a passageway or the centre of a room or by bringing a stronger beam of light on to the area where you are sewing, reading or working.

When you are twenty years old it is often possible to do fine tasks such as reading or sewing without a good light source, but the older you get, the more difficult this becomes. Maximum light can be obtained by bringing a standard lamp, table lamp or reading lamp close to where you are sitting, working or reading so that the beam falls directly on to the object you are looking at. Similarly, if you have always used a lamp at the side of the chair where you read, put in a stronger bulb. Stronger light in passageways, halls and stairs can also reduce the risk of falling.

Regular Eye Testing

Most people over the age of sixty need glasses for a least some tasks and some people have to wear glasses all the time. Because the eye is changing as we age, it is as important to have regular vision checks in old age as in youth. You should have your eyes tested at least once every two years, but you may need more frequent tests and you should always go to an optician if you notice that your vision is failing.

You can have your eyes tested either by an optician or in one of the new stores specializing in spectacles. If you have your eyes tested in a specialist shop, you will certainly have the services of an optician to test your eyes, but you may come under tougher pressure to buy a new pair of glasses from one of the sales staff.

Although your eyes are changing all the time, the change may not be a significant one, but it may be hard for you to judge how great it actually is. One way to assess this is to ask the optician if you can try your old glasses on again after they have completed making up the right lenses for you in the special frames that are used during eye testing. What usually happens is that you take your glasses off, have your eyes tested, and at the end of the test you are able to see the test board clearly because of the combination of lenses that have been put into the special testing frame. The end result is obviously clearer than the blurred view of the letters on the chart that you had when the test started, but is is not necessarily much clearer than the view that you would get with your old spectacles on. So, before leaving your seat, say to the optician, 'Now that you have prepared the new lenses for me I would just like to look through my old glasses to see if there is much of a difference.' If you notice a significant difference between your old glasses and the proposed new lenses, it is wise to have a new pair of glasses made up because glasses that do not give clear focus can cause headaches and difficulties with carrying out tasks that require good vision.

Difficulty with Hearing

Normal ageing reduces your ability to hear high notes. For most people this causes no problem at all because it is only the highest notes that cannot be heard.

A simple experiment can demonstrate this to you. All you need for this experiment is a youngster – your grandchild or some other young person – and something that can make a very high note – a piano, or a child's xylophone or triangle will do. Explain to the child that you would like her help with an experiment. Ask her to hold her hand above her head and then with the other hand make or play the highest musical note she can. Say that when she stops hearing the note she can bring her hand down and that you will hold your hand above your head and bring it down too when you can no longer hear the sound of the note. Now ask the youngster to play the high note and see what happens.

Almost always the young person's hand stays up longer than the hand of the older person because the latter loses the ability to hear high notes. For most people this causes no problem at all until very old age – that is, over ninety. The reason for this is that we do not need to hear the very high notes very often in modern life, and most people can continue to hear the phone and take part in normal conversation until their late eighties or nineties.

Why Do Some People Become Deaf?

Deafness is due to a disease and not to normal ageing. There are a number of different diseases, which can cause loss of hearing, not all of which are clearly understood, but the effects of most are similar.

When Does Hearing Loss Become a Problem?

The answer to this one is simple: hearing loss becomes a problem when you *feel* it is a problem, either because you notice it interfering with your everyday life or because of the fact that you are anxious about what might happen in the future.

If you are worried about loss of hearing, see your doctor who will be able to check for some of the causes. One of these is wax in the ears, which the doctor may wash out or ask the practice nurse to do so. If you have had wax in the ears before and suspect that it is again the cause of your hearing problems, try to soften the wax yourself – for example by dropping warm olive oil into the affected ear. Put some warm oil on a teaspoon and just let it drop into the ear. Do not attempt to put any object into the ear or you may damage it.

If your hearing loss is not due to wax in the ear, there is little that your GP can do himself or herself to help, but he or she can refer you to the ear, nose and throat department of your local hospital for assessment.

Should I Approach a Company That Sells Hearing Aids?

The Yellow Pages lists a number of suppliers of hearing aids and they often advertise in newspapers and magazines. Some of the aids that can be purchased are better than those which are available on the National Health Service, but not all hearing aid suppliers are equally dependable. It is, therefore, important to seek expert advice before buying.

What if my General Practitioner Isn't Helpful?

If your GP does not suggest going for a hearing test, you can suggest it yourself. The simplest way to do this would be to say, 'I am thinking of buying a hearing aid, and I am told it is best to have your hearing checked by the hospital first. Could you refer me to the clinic please?' If the doctor is still unhelpful, you can contact your local voluntary association concerned with the problems of deaf people. Even though they are usually concerned principally with people who are completely deaf, they are often able to give very sensible advice to those who are hard of hearing (including, in the case of the Royal National Institute for the Deaf, printed material about hearing aids). You will find these organizations, under 'Deaf' in the phone book.

How Can I Help Other People?

Your problem may be that someone else close to you is becoming hard of hearing. If they are not prepared to admit it, life can be difficult for both of you, but if you can keep your temper and not get irritated with the other person's hearing difficulties, they will usually admit they have a problem and seek help.

In speaking to someone who is hard of hearing there are a few simple tips that should be remembered:

- Speak slowly rather than loudly; shouting is not helpful and simply annoys the person who is hard of hearing.
- Make sure that the person who is hard of hearing can see your face clearly – for example, by sitting

so that your face is in the light when speaking to them, and by keeping your face turned towards them all the time.

- Don't try to exaggerate lip movements when talking to a person who is hard of hearing.
- Make sure that background noise such as a radio or television is kept to a minimum.
- Remember that people who are hard of hearing may be embarrassed about their problem and may need special help at social gatherings. For instance, at a party it may be difficult for the deaf person to hear another speaking; if this is the case, help them find a quite corner so that they can listen to another person speaking in comfort.

There are a number of electrical appliances which can help deaf people to use the telephone, hear the doorbell or the television. Ask the health visitors (see page 68), or enquire at the ear, nose and throat department of your local hospital or at the nearest deaf centre for further information about these.

Finding Hidden Health Problems

There was a fashion ten or twenty years ago for encouraging people to have regular health checks, rather like giving a car annual MOT tests. The idea was that you took your body to the doctor every six months or every year and the doctor looked at it and in it and did some tests on it and then did some things to reduce the risk of disease or improve your health.

However, enthusiasm for routine health testing died away in the 1970s and early 1980s because many people discovered that regular health testing, in a way like taking a car to a garage for regular servicing, does not necessarily lead to better health. In fact, some people find that taking their car to the garage for a regular check can result in its running less well than before it went in.

There are, though, a number of diseases which do go through a phase in their development before they become obvious to you. This is sometimes called the pre-clinical phase because it is the period before they become clinically obvious by causing symptoms that you feel, or signs that the doctor can detect. For some of these diseases it is possible to detect the pre-clinical phase by special tests, but finding a disease early does not always lead to its cure. Sometimes early detection of a disease leads to longer survival of the patients, but longer survival does not necessarily mean that the test produced a cure.

Imagine that there is a type of cancer which takes six years from its origin to the moment when it becomes fatal, and that it has a pre-clinical period of three years before it causes signs and symptoms which take the person with the cancer to the doctor. If a test is introduced which detects that cancer one year after it starts growing, the survival after detection might be five years, compared with three years after the onset of signs and symptoms at the beginning of the clinical phase. Thus the test appears to increase survival by two years but in fact it simply allows the person to know five years rather than three years in advance that they are going to die, and some people would prefer not to have these extra years' knowledge if there was no increase in actual survival time.

For this reason doctors are very cautious about tests for hidden disease, called screening tests, and there are just three which can be recommended to all older people, the first two for women only:

1 The cervical smear test for changes which might develop into cancer of the cervix.
2 Mammography for breast cancer.
3 Blood pressure measurement for the detection of high blood pressure.

The Cervical Smear Test

The cervix is the part of the uterus (womb) where it is joined on to the vagina. The cells covering the cervix and lining the passage through the cervix into the uterus can become cancerous. The cervical smear test can detect changes in blood cells before they become cancerous, enabling treatment to be given at the pre-cancerous stage of this disease, which is most common among older women.

The cervical smear test is for all women, but women who have never had sexual intercourse are at very very low risk of cervical cancer, and it is not usual to offer the test to this group. If you have never had a cervical smear test, you should ask if you can have one done (see page 57). If you are over sixty-five and had had at least one normal cervical smear test, you are at a low risk of cervical cancer and probably do not need another smear test; if you have had two or more normal smear tests, you are at a very low risk of cervical cancer indeed.

To do the cervical smear test the doctor does an internal examination and then inserts a metal or plastic instrument called a speculum into the vagina. This allows the doctor to look at the cervix and scrape a sample of cells off its surface. These are then smeared on to a glass slide which is sent to the laboratory for examination under a microscope.

The test should not be painful but it is sometimes very uncomfortable for older women because the tissues of the vagina change after the menopause and make the test more difficult than it is in younger women. It is also more difficult for the doctor to do the test after the menopause because the number of cells that can be obtained is reduced.

The cervical smear test is not a test for cancer. It is a test for pre-cancer, for changes in the cervix that might become cancer if left untreated. If you are told that you need another smear test, this does not mean that you have cancer; it may simply mean that there were not enough cells on the smear for the laboratory staff to read the smear, or it may mean that you are at a slightly higher risk of cancer than average and need a follow-up. A small number of women are referred for colposcopy. The colposcope is something which allows a doctor to examine your cervix closely when he or she is doing an internal examination. Colposcopy is an outpatient procedure which does not require general anaesthetic.

Mammography for Breast Cancer
A woman should *always* see her doctor *as soon as* she notices any kind of change in the appearance of a breast, or a lump in the breast, or a discharge from the nipple, because any of these can mean that she has cancer. While it should be remembered that not all lumps are cancerous, it is vital to have them checked immediately.

The best way to reduce the mortality for breast cancer, which is still the commonest cancer among women in Britain, is to detect the disease at a much earlier stage in its development. Mammography can do this.

Mammography is an X-ray picture taken of breast

tissue. It allows the detection of cancers which are too small to be felt as lumps but which usually, though not always, show up on the X-ray. If you have not had a mammogram in the previous three years, you need the test.

Mammography takes about half an hour. The woman is asked to undress and an X-ray picture is taken of each breast in turn. The breast is placed on a flat surface with a rounded edge and a plastic surface is gently but firmly brought down on top of the breast. An X-ray picture is taken and the procedure is then repeated with the other breast. Taking the mammogram itself is very quick, but dressing and undressing, filling out your form and getting information about the mammography add up to the rest of the thirty minutes.

About 10% of women who have a mammogram are told that they need another test, and this causes a good deal of unnecessary anxiety as only a very small proportion of these people actually have cancer. Sometimes the film needs to be repeated, simply because the first film was not of a good enough quality to allow the person examining it to reach a definite decision. Sometimes additional films are needed or other tests (which are painless) are used to help the doctor to decide whether something seen in the X-ray is actually cancer or whether there is a type of breast disease which is not cancer.

Before the diagnosis of cancer is actually made, it is necessary to have a biopsy. This is an operation requiring general anaesthetic which requires an overnight stay in hospital. The doctor removes a small piece of breast tissue, called a biopsy, and this is examined under a microscope by a pathologist.

Remember that, even if you have had a mammogram, you must continue to be alert to changes in the appearance of your breasts, and if you notice a change in the appearance of a breast, or a discharge from a nipple, or a lump, you should go to see your doctor as soon as possible.

Finding Cancer Early

The two cancer screening tests described above help detect the disease before it becomes obvious. However, it is also important to be aware of some of the other early signs of cancer and to seek help when these occur. In many cases these symptoms do not indicate that the person has cancer, but they can be early warning signs and should never be ignored:

- Persistent hoarseness lasting for three weeks or more.
- Any mole or swelling on your skin which changes in appearance or size or becomes tender.
- Passage of blood from the vagina, or while you are passing water, or from the back passage.
- Any swelling or lump that you notice in your abdomen.
- Any alteration in bowel habits, particularly alternating constipation and diarrhoea.

Measuring Blood Pressure

Everyone who is alive has blood pressure. It is blood pressure that drives blood round your circulatory system in the same way that water pressure drives the water round your central heating system at home. If, however, the pressure is too high, it increases the risk of a stroke, and if the blood pressure is very much higher than average, reducing it by use of medicines reduces the risk of a stroke.

You have almost certainly had your blood pressure measured at least once in you life, and perhaps on many occasions. To take the measurement an instrument called a sphygmomanometer is used. Everyone needs a blood pressure measurement at least once every five years up to the age of seventy-five. After that age there is little evidence that the treatment of high blood pressure lowers the risk of a stroke. Doctors do not usually go looking for high blood pressure in people over seventy-five, but if someone has reached that age and has been on treatment for a number of years, their doctor may decide to continue the treatment depending upon the height of the person's blood pressure and how well they feel on the treatment.

If you are under seventy-five and cannot remember having had your blood pressure measured in the last five years, you need to have it measured. If you have had your blood pressure measured in the last five years and it was at a satisfactory level, you do not need another test until five years are up. If you are receiving treatment for high blood pressure, you need to see your doctor at least once every six months or every year, depending upon your level of blood pressure and how well your treatment is working. The doctor will measure your blood pressure and may carry out other tests, such as on the blood or urine, when you go for these check-ups.

The higher your blood pressure, the higher the risk of a stroke, but your doctor has to balance the possible benefits of giving you treatment with the problems that can occur from taking drugs to lower your blood pressure because these drugs sometimes have side effects. The decision to start treatment is made in much the same way as you decide to replace the tyres on a car. You cannot be sure that you would have a crash if you did not replace the tyres and you may still have a crash on a wet road even with new tyres, but replacing old and bald car tyres with new ones reduces the risk of a crash and most people think it is worth the expense to do this. It is the same with deciding whether or not to start treatment for high blood pressure. It does involve some difficulty, but it does reduce the risk of a stroke.

How Can I Get these Screening Tests?
You can have your blood pressure measured, or a cervical smear test carried out, by your own doctor. Simply explain to the receptionist what you require and ask if it is possible to make an appointment to see your doctor or the practice nurse.

Your own doctor cannot do mammography, which is carried out by a special X-ray machine situated in a screening centre, or hospital or a mobile X-ray clinic. Between 1988 and 1990 breast cancer screening services will be introduced throughout the UK. If you are aged fifty to sixty-four, your local service will obtain your address from your GP's list and issue an invitation to you by post to have a test once every three years. If you are sixty-five or over but would like a test, ask your doctor's receptionist to make an appointment for you to discuss mammography with the doctor, or to ask the doctor if he or she will make an appointment for you to have the test.

Your doctor's receptionist should have information about these screening tests but if you would like more information and cannot get it from your own GP, write to the addresses below. Information about the prevention of stroke and heart disease may be obtained from: The Chest, Heart and Stroke Association, Tavistock House, North Tavistock Square, London WC1. Information about cancer may be obtained from: The Women's National Cancer Control Campaign, 1 South Audley Street, London W1.

The Ageing Skin

Changes in the skin and hair are the most obvious signs of ageing and much time and money is spent on attempts to minimize these effects.

The skin consists of approximately twenty layers of cells and is about the thickness of a sheet of writing paper. Underneath this is the fibrous tissue containing blood vessels which nourishes the skin. As with so many aspect of body ageing, it is difficult to distinguish the effects of the normal biological ageing process from the effects of social or environmental changes, and it is now known that many of the changes in the skin that were formerly thought to be due to ageing are in fact due to exposure to sun and, to a lesser extent, wind.

In the deepest cell layers there are pigment cells which protect the body against sunlight. These cells are progressively lost with age, so the older you are, the more sensitive to sunlight is your skin. Not only do the pigment cells generally decrease in numbers as you age, but in some parts of the skin they increase in a localized patch giving rise to the large freckles, sometimes called 'age spots', which can be seen, for example, on the back of the hands of many older people.

The best means of slowing down the change in the appearance of the skin is to minimize its exposure to sunlight. Try to stick to the following rules:

- If you want a tan, go for a light one rather than a deep tan.
- Use sunblocking cream whenever possible – the better the protection from ultraviolet light, the better for your skin.

- Expose as little of your body as possible to the sun; if you wish to keep your face looking as young as possible, expose it to the sun as little as you can.

Many products are advertised in a way that implies that they delay or reverse skin ageing, but the scientific facts are not very encouraging. Moisturizers can help people with dry skin look and feel better, but don't actually have any effect on the ageing process, neither do products which contain oestrogen. So the main message therefore remains the simple one already quoted: to slow down the ageing of the skin, reduce exposure to sunlight.

Health Problems Arising from Too Much Sunlight on the Skin

As well as speeding up the ageing of the skin, too much sunlight can actually endanger your health in other ways than the obvious one of causing sunstroke. Sunlight is known to be linked with skin cancer, of which there are three common types – a squamous cancer which may appear as a skin ulcer anywhere on the body; a basal cell cancer (sometimes called rodent ulcer) which usually appears on the face; and melanoma, a mole which changes to cancer. All three types are seen more frequently in people who have a long history of exposure to the sun. Because these cancers are on the surface of the skin, they can be diagnosed early, and it is important to go to your doctor if you:

- Have a cut or sore that does not heal easily.
- Notice a mole or brown spot changing in shape or appearance, or becoming ulcerated.

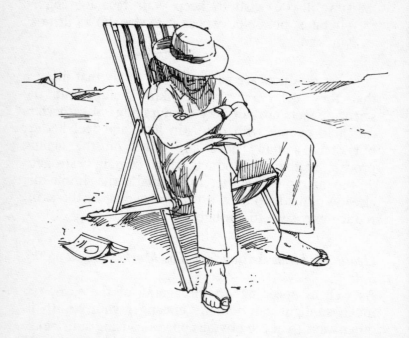

Does Sunlight Have Any Benefit?
It is necessary to expose the skin to some sunlight
because this stimulates it to manufacture vitamin D,
which plays an important part in the prevention of
bone disease (osteomalacia) in old age. Therefore you
should *not* try to keep out of the sun altogether but,
because of the dangers outlined above, bare your skin
to its rays only with caution. It seems that you can
make enough vitamin D to see you through the
winter by getting a good tan on your forearms and
upper arms, such as can be achieved by wearing a
short-sleeved shirt, while at the same time protecting
your face, not only to reduce the skin cancer of this
vulnerable area but also to keep the skin on your face
looking as young as possible.

What Can Be Done about Skin Disease in Old Age?

Because of the ageing process, the effect of sunlight and, for many people, the effects of decades of exposure of the skin to dust, dirt, cosmetics, detergents, water, or a combination of all these factors, many older people develop skin problems or notice that the skin problems that they have had for years become worse. In addition, some people develop ulcers in the skin, particularly on the lower part of the leg. These leg (or varicose) ulcers may be associated with obvious varicose veins, or may be caused by underlying problems with the veins which are not obvious on the surface.

It is important not to try treating skin disease yourself other than by applying a moisturiser in the case of dry skin. The skin becomes more sensitive as it ages, and sometimes you can actually make skin disease worse by attempting home treatment if your skin develops a sensitivity to one of the chemicals in the ointment or cream you are using. This is not an allergy in the true sense of the word but rather a chemical sensitivity.

If your doctor cannot solve your skin problems, he or she can make a referral to a hospital specialist, called a dermatologist. If you develop a leg ulcer, the doctor will probably ask the practice nurse or district nurse to supervise treatment.

7 SERVICES: YOUR OPPORTUNITIES AND RIGHTS

There are a large number of services available to help people with problems. Not all of them work as well in one part of the country as they do in another, and you can even find quite marked differences between one health centre and another or even between one professional and another. For example, one social worker appears to be competent and efficient, while another may appear to be less helpful to an older person. These variations in quality of care are inevitable, although they need not be as great as they are at present when individuals seeking help often have to overcome obstacles to obtain the help to which they are entitled. The objective of this chapter is to outline ways in which you can get the best out of the services available.

The General Practitioner

One of the most important professionals in the life of a retired person is the general practitioner, or family doctor. If you need to find a doctor, perhaps because you have moved house, ask as many people as possible if they would recommend their own GP.

Don't just rely on one opinion, because someone may dislike a doctor who is actually very good while another person may think very highly of a doctor who is generally thought to be mediocre. The more people you ask, the better picture you will get.

Before you make a decision, consider other important factors, such as the ease with which you can reach your prospective doctor's health centre or surgery. Write to the GP you have in mind and ask if he or she will accept you as a patient. If he or she is unable to do so, write to your second choice.

Working with Your General Practitioner

Your doctor and you are in partnership – a partnership for health. There are three different types of occasion on which you will need help from your doctor: when you need regular health checks, when you need treatment for chronic disease and when you suddenly feel unwell.

REGULAR HEALTH CHECKS

There is no need to have regular health checks if you are feeling well and healthy, but there are three tests that can detect hidden disease which your doctor can provide or arrange for you: the cervical smear test, mammography for early breast cancer, and the measurement of your blood pressure. These are described on page 50.

TREATMENT FOR CHRONIC DISEASE

When you have a chronic or long-standing health problem, your doctor is able to help you in a number of ways by treating the disease itself, by helping you cope with the changes that result from that disease, by suggesting things you can do to make the problem less of a burden and, when necessary, by referring you to hospital. Of all the things that the doctor can do, two are of particular importance – treating you safely and effectively with drugs and referring you to hospital when appropriate.

Medicines bring many benefits to older people, but they can also cause problems because they often have side effects. For this reason some older people stop taking the medicines that they were prescribed. Here are a few simple rules to remember if you are taking medicines or repeat prescriptions:

1 Don't stop taking your medicine merely because you think it is not working, or because you think it is having side effects, without seeking advice from the pharmacist who dispensed the medicine or the doctor who prescribed it.

2 If you think that your medicine is making you feel unwell, contact either the pharmacist or your doctor as soon as you can to seek advice.

3 Find ways of remembering to take your medicine as frequently as it was prescribed – for example, by always taking it with meals or when you get up. If you have not remembered to take it as often as you should have done, tell the doctor when you next see him or her.

4 If you have been taking medicine for more than a year without seeing your doctor, you should make an appointment to see if he or she is happy with your progress.

GPs make hundreds of thousands of referrals to hospital each year, but from the patient's point of view the most important time comes when he or she has lost confidence in the doctor's opinion, or thinks that a second opinion might be helpful. It is obviously difficult to raise this with your doctor because it suggests that you have lost faith in his or her ability, but most GPs know that when people become anxious about disease they want to try every possible avenue to improve their health. The simplest way to approach the problem is simply to say to your doctor, 'I know you have done everything you can but I just wondered if there is any test or treatment that only the hospital could provide which could help me. Do you think you could refer me to hospital to see if something could be done there?' This makes it clear that you would like a referral not simply because you think hospital doctors are better able to diagnose or treat than GPs but because you know that they have many more resources in hospital.

WHEN YOU SUDDENLY FEEL UNWELL

The third type of occasion when people seek help from their GP is when they feel unwell, and when this is the case you have to decide whether you want a home visit or whether you can reach the surgery, and if it is a surgery appointment how quickly you want that appointment.

Usually you will have to ask the receptionist whether the doctor can call at your home, she will have been told to try to encourage as many people as possible to go to the surgery. This is not because the doctor is lazy or dislikes home visiting, but because he or she is able to help more people by seeing as many as possible at the surgery – four or five people in the time it takes to make one home visit, and this problem is getting worse as traffic and parking gets more difficult. If you really feel that you cannot get to the surgery, just say to the receptionist, 'I really feel too unwell to drive or even be driven and would like a home visit. If you like, I could explain to the doctor myself how unwell I am feeling.' You then may be able to phone the doctor at a time that is convenient to him or her – for example, during coffee after morning surgery – and explain then why you would appreciate a home visit.

If the decision is that you should go to the surgery, the receptionist needs to decide how quickly she can fit you in. Almost all doctors try to see people who are acutely ill quickly, but they can only do this if patients whose problems are less acute are willing to accept appointments a week or two in advance. One way in which the receptionist can judge this is by asking how long your problem has lasted. If it has lasted for months already, you can probably wait a bit longer. If, on the other hand, it has only blown up in the last day or two, you may need to be seen quickly.

How to Change Your Doctor?

Sometimes you may decide that you just want to change your doctor completely and the following steps can help you do so:

1 Find the name of another GP who would be suitable by asking as many of your friends as possible for a recommendation.
2 Write to that doctor to ask if he or she will accept you as a patient. An explanation or reason why you want to change from one practice to another may be helpful, but is not necessary.
3 If the doctor is willing to accept you on to his or her list, either inform the receptionist at your present health centre, in writing or in person, that you are being transferred to the list of the new doctor, or write directly to your local Family Practitioner Committee and ask them to arrange a transfer.

Each GP is a member not only of a partnership but also of a team, sometimes called the primary care team. The other members of this team are the district nurse, the health visitor and the practice nurse.

The District Nurse

The district nurse specializes in the provision of specialist nursing care for people in their own homes. The type of special nursing that she has to offer is demonstrated by the following list of tasks which are usually performed by district nurses:

- The treatment of leg ulcers.
- Insulin injections for people who are blind and thus cannot inject themselves.
- The assessment of people who have suddenly become disabled – for example, as the result of a stroke – and the provision of intensive nursing during the early phase of recovery.
- General care: for example, bathing is done in some parts of the country by nursing auxiliaries who work for district nurses, but in other parts of the country this type of work is done by care assistants working for the Social Services Department.

To contact the district nurse phone the health centre and ask if you can speak to her or if she can phone you. You do not need to speak to the doctor before making contact with the district nurse.

The Health Visitor

The health visitor is a nurse with a special training in prevention. Most of her work is with mothers and babies, but health visiting has an interest in preventing the problems of old age, and some health visitors spend quite a bit of their time helping people as they age. The health visitor is specially trained and able to give advice to individuals or groups; if you were, for instance, the secretary of a parish council or a voluntary organization and wanted to know how best your organization could help older people, she would be the ideal person to advise you.

You can contact the health visitor by phoning your surgery or health centre and asking how you can get in touch with her. You do not need to speak to the doctor before contacting the health visitor.

The Practice Nurse

An increasing number of medical practices employ nurses who work in the health centre. The type of tasks that they carry out include: washing out wax from the ears; the treatment of leg ulcers; immunizations for flu or foreign travel; and follow-up checks for people with diabetes or high blood pressure.

You could ask your doctor if you think a practice nurse could help you, but usually the suggestion comes from the doctor.

The Social Services Department

The Social Services Department (in Scotland called the Social Work Department) provides a wide range of services; only the more important are discussed in this section. Each Department can supply information about its own services and the staff are usually knowledgeable about social security benefits. (Alternative sources of help are the Citizens Advice Bureaux and Housing Aid Centres.)

The Social Worker

The social worker is usually seen as someone who arranges things for others, such as an admission to an old people's home or the provision of some service. However, the real job of the social worker is to help individuals and families sort out and solve problems that they cannot tackle successfully without the help of an outsider, as the following example illustrates.

Mrs W is sixty-two; her mother is ninety-four and soon ready to be discharged from hospital following a stroke. The old lady says she wants to return to her own home, but Mrs W feels that she should have her mother to stay with her, partly because she is anxious and partly because she feels guilty that she has done so little for her mother in the past. Mr W does not like Mrs W's mother – one of the reasons why Mrs W has done so little over the years – and says that if her mother comes to stay he will move out. The Ws have a daughter who is getting divorced and wants to come back to live with her parents. The job of the social worker is to help Mr and Mrs W and the others involved in this family tangle to reach an acceptable solution to their problems – probably by helping Mrs W's mother with enough support to remain at home and helping Mrs W cope with the anxiety and guilt that she will feel as a result, even though she agrees that this may be the best for all concerned.

To contact a social worker, phone or call in at the local Social Services Department and ask for an appointment.

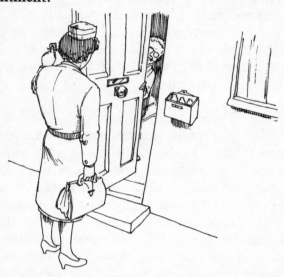

Support Services
Social Services Departments organize and provide home help services for those who cannot do their own housework or shopping; meals on wheels for those who have difficulty in buying and/or preparing food; home care for those people who need the type of practical assistance with dressing or bathing that would be provided by a healthy middle-aged child if they had one living near who was willing to provide such help. In many parts of the country these services are very limited and your doctor or district nurse may be able to advise you on how best to obtain support for yourself or for your parent.

8 COMMON HEALTH PROBLEMS IN OLD AGE

There is not enough space within this book to cover all the health problems that can occur in old age, and indeed there are already good books available on common health problems for people of all ages. The Reader's Digest *Family Medical Adviser*, for example, provides a useful summary of many common conditions and diseases, and explains in simple language terms used by doctors such as electro-cardiogram (ECG), or diuretic. This chapter focuses principally on those health problems to which older people and their relatives need to pay particular attention, either when consulting such a reference book or when deciding whether or not to contact their doctor.

There are two important questions that you have to answer when things go wrong with your health in old age. The first, when you initially notice something amiss, is simply, 'Is this part of old age that I have to accept, or could my doctor do something about it?' The second question, which arises when you know you have a problem that cannot be cured, is, 'How can I best adapt to this problem so that it interferes with my life as little as possible?' Let us consider each of these questions, in turn.

Is this part of old age that I have to accept, or could my doctor do something about it?

As you grow older health problems become more common, and it is not unusual to notice an ache in one part of the body or another, or to feel tired and weak or to notice that you are out of breath after climbing a couple of flights of stairs or going up a hill. These changes are often temporary and clear up by themselves. If, however, you notice something wrong with you that does not clear up, you need to seek advice, and the best person to consult is your GP.

It is often hard to distinguish the effects of normal ageing from the effects of disease, either in yourself or in someone else whom you visit or see from time to time. When should you decide to consult a doctor about a problem that has been coming on over a few months or weeks? Bear in mind that the effects of the ageing process tend to be very slow and take place over months or years, whereas the effects of disease usually take place over a shorter period of time. Some problems, such as a stroke, develop all of a sudden; others over the course of a day or two, and it is usually quite easy to spot such health problems and seek help from a doctor. When the change comes on more slowly, however, over a period of week or months, it can be difficult to decide if you just have to accept the feeling of, say, tiredness or breathlessness as part of old age, or if you should visit your GP and ask him or her to examine you to see if a treatable, and perhaps curable, cause for your problem can be found.

The following guidelines may help you make this decision:

• The more quickly a problem has come on, the more likely is it to be due to a disease.

- If someone you have not seen for some time comments that you are not looking as well as you did when they last saw you, you should ask yourself if you have been keeping well and possibly see your doctor – a person who is falling ill is sometimes the last to notice the change that has taken place in himself or herself.

- If a health problem is interfering with your ability to look after yourself or get out and enjoy yourself, you should consult the doctor; normal ageing does not usually affect the quality of life and the ability of individuals to look after themselves until they reach an advanced age of ninety or over.

- If you are worried about your health problem, you should see your doctor. For example, many people notice that they are getting forgetful and are worried that this is the first sign of Alzheimer's disease, or senile dementia; and it can be very reassuring to be told that normal ageing and not the onset of a serious disease is the cause of these minor slips in memory.

How can I best adapt to this problem so that it interferes with my life as little as possible?

Some diseases are completely curable but many that occur in old age are not. These, known as chronic diseases, last a long period of time – sometimes as long as the person lives. Do not be afraid to ask for help from NHS employees when you are struggling to adapt to life with a chronic disease. It is primarily the doctor's job to diagnose and treat disease, and in the case of chronic problems such as incontinence or leg ulcers (which may be caused by a number of different diseases), it is often the district nurse (see page 67) who has more to do with helping people cope with distressing symptoms. Disabilities such as difficulty with dressing or getting about inside or outside the house are obviously of importance to doctors and nurses, but physiotherapists and occupational therapists are the people to turn to for help in this area. However, there are very few occupational therapists or physiotherapists working outside hospitals, so in fact the GP often has to help people who are disabled.

Common Chronic Diseases

Common chronic diseases that occur in old age are: bronchitis, various types of heart disease, diabetes, arthritis, high blood pressure, psychological problems (such as depression and anxiety), Alzheimer's disease and stroke. The following guidelines are intended to help you if you suffer from a chronic disease:

● **Be confident in the medical advice you are receiving**. Obviously you cannot know everything about a disease that a doctor knows, but you have to be confident that the doctor has the diagnosis correct, has done all the tests that should be done and is giving you the best possible treatment. If you are not confident, you should consider asking the doctor for a second opinion – that is, a referral to hospital. People find this a difficult topic to discuss with their GP because they do not like to give him or her the impression that they have lost trust, but many GPs would prefer patients to be honest and say if they want a second opinion rather than visiting the surgery on numerous occasions because they are not certain that they are getting the best treatment possible.

Sometimes other people say things that make you

think you should be referred. A friend may tell you about a relative who was referred to hospital with a disease like yours and who is getting treatment that you are not receiving, or you may read in the papers or see reports on television about treatments which you are not being offered. Often the press gives a false impression of what treatments are best for a condition because journalists usually concentrate on the most advanced treatments which may still be at an experimental stage. If, however, you are wondering whether such a treatment or test would help you, the best thing is simply to ask your GP. Make an appointment to see him or her and when you go in and the doctor asks 'How are you getting on?' say what is in your mind – for example, 'Well, I'm not doing too badly, but I read about this new treatment for my condition, and I wonder whether the treatment is available at the local hospital and whether you could refer me to see if it is suitable for me.'

Similarly, if you just feel that you are not making the progress that you think you should be making, you could say to the doctor, 'I am very grateful for what you have done to try to help me, doctor, but I am getting depressed about my condition and I wonder if you could refer me to hospital to see if anything more could be done?' (See also pages 64–5.)

● **Take the treatment the doctor has prescribed for you**. The most common reason why people do not take medicine in the way the doctor prescribes it is that the doctor does not give clear enough advice about the way in which he or she wants the medicine to be taken. If you are in any doubt at all about the best way to take the medicine prescribed for you, ask the pharmacist who dispenses your prescription.

Pharmacists know a great deal about medicines, their side effects and actions, and the best way to take them. Ask at the chemist if you do not know precisely what you are meant to do with your prescription.

If you feel that the medicine is not having any effect, carry on taking it until you can see the doctor again to tell him or her. You must remember that not all medicines have effects you can feel, and even though you don't feel any change in your state of health the medicine may still be doing you good – for example, by reducing the risk of a complication.

Similarly, if you think that the medicine you have been prescribed is making you feel unwell, do not simply stop taking it. If you cannot speak to the doctor who gave you the prescription, ask at the chemist's shop. Explain the health problems that you think has been caused by the medicine that you have recently started taking, and ask the chemist if he or she thinks that you should carry on taking it.

● **Make sure that you get as much information as you want**.   Almost always people want to know more about the disease they have than their doctor tells them. If you want to know more, you could say to your doctor, 'I don't want to take up any more of your time now, doctor, but can you give me something more to read about my problem or recommend me a book to buy or somewhere I can write for more information?' Oxford University Press produces a very good series of books about common health problems called 'The Facts' (obtainable from most bookshops.)

If a doctor cannot give you the information you need, ask the health visitor (see page 68) or enquire at your local community health council. There is now a society for most chronic diseases to which sufferers and their relatives can turn to for further information and advice: again, your local community health council will give you details.

● **Share your cares**. As well as information, people with health problems need sympathy and support. Sometimes the support comes naturally from the doctors and nurses involved, and from friends and relations, but this does not always happen. If you feel that you have not really had an opportunity to speak to anyone about your problem and the effect that it has had on your life, you should try to find someone to share your cares with. The sort of feelings in a patient that doctors sometimes overlook is that what has happened is not fair, and it is important to talk to someone if you feel angry about developing an illness, because if you become bitter with the suffering of your illness it will be all the more difficult to bear. The following case illustrates this point.

Mrs A's husband developed a rare form of Parkinson's disease soon after retirement. He seemed to adapt well to the problems that the disease caused, but Mrs A thought repeatedly, 'It doesn't seem right; he has led a good life and is entitled to enjoy his retirement, and now this happens.' The impact of Parkinson's disease on the life of Mr and Mrs A was greatly activated by these feelings which were turning to bitterness until they made an appointment to see the medical social worker at the hospital where Mr A was attending out patient clinics. They were able to have a long talk about the illness, and its effect on their life and marriage, which has helped Mrs A to come to terms with her husband's condition.

Some people are simply puzzled by the fact that diseases happen to them and spend a lot of time wondering, 'Why me? Why am I suffering when others are spared?' Your GP is in the best position to help you deal with this sort of feeling, but not all people get on well enough with their doctor to be able to discuss such an issue with him or her. Other people you can turn to for help include the district nurse or health visitor who is working with your GP (see pages 67 and 68): nurses are often able to speak to people suffering from disease about this type of problem more easily than doctors. If you are going to hospital either as an in patient or an out patient, you could ask for an appointment at the medical social work department of the hospital, like Mr and Mrs A in the case described above. You may also be able to find great support from making contact with the society or association dedicated to helping people with your condition.

● **Keep in touch with your doctor**. If you are suffering from a chronic disease, it is essential that you keep in touch with your doctor, particularly if you are taking medicines regularly. If you are taking medicines which require repeat prescriptions, you should see your doctor at least once every six months and sometimes more frequently than that. If you have been taking medicines for more than six months without seeing your doctor, you should make an appointment to see him or her, and when the doctor asks the reason for the appointment simply say, 'I have been worrying about my condition and really just came to check up that everything is going well.'

● **Be positive: set yourself targets**. When you have a chronic health problem, you have to fight it. Try to identify small steps you can take to overcome even a part of your problem. If, for example, you feel that life is not worth living, write down the three things that bother you most and see if your doctor or nurse can help you tackle them.

Coping with Chronic Diseases
As has already been mentioned, it is not possible to describe in this book the diseases that commonly occur in old age, but there are one or two points that you should always remember if you or a friend or a relative develops any of these common diseases.

BRONCHITIS
Whatever the cause of your lung disease, you will feel better and be fitter if you manage to give up smoking (see page 26). You might also be helped by influenza immunization, so make a note about this in your diary on 1 October and when that date arrives ask your doctor if he or she thinks that you will benefit from it.

HEART DISEASE
If you have heart disease, you should try to help yourself by:

- Giving up smoking (see page 26).
- Losing weight (see page 20).

In addition your doctor may recommend that you take a small dose of aspirin every day to stop your blood clotting.

DIABETES
There are three important things you can do to help yourself if you develop diabetes:

- Stop smoking (see page 26).
- Take more exercise (see pages 31–40).
- Lose weight (see page 20).

ARTHRITIS
If you feel that your arthritis is getting worse or if the drugs your doctor has prescribed are causing you pain, you can ask your doctor to refer you to a consultant rheumatologist. Keeping fit and getting fitter help you cope with arthritis by reducing stiffness and increasing muscle strength.

DEPRESSION AND ANXIETY
Everyone feels depressed or anxious from time to time, but you should go to see your doctor if:

- You can't stop thinking about your problem.
- You have tried speaking about your worries to friends, relatives and people you trust, but still feel anxious or depressed.
- You cannot get to sleep at night or wake up early thinking about your problem.
- You cannot speak to people properly because the topic you are worried or depressed about keeps breaking into your thoughts.
- You ever think of suicide as a means of solving your problem.

Remember that the medication used for the treatment of anxiety and depression can have side effects in old age, and you should ask your doctor if there are other steps you could take to deal with your problem. You may find that the following steps help in helping you cope with anxiety or depression:

1 Tackle the cause and try to solve it.
2 If you cannot identify one specific cause, write down the things that seem to make you most anxious or depressed and try to tackle them.
3 Share your thoughts and feelings with someone else; speak to anyone whose opinion you trust if you do not find your doctor easy to talk to.
4 Try to change your lifestyle in two ways: for example, by changing your diet, or by taking more exercise, or by taking up a new hobby.
5 Try to meet other people more frequently than you do at present.

ALZHEIMER'S DISEASE

You will probably not be reading this book if you are developing Alzheimer's disease because failure of intellectual ability is one of the first signs, but you may notice this in somebody else. However, there are a number of other causes of slowly developing confusion in old age. If someone you know becomes noticeably more forgetful, it is important that their doctor examines them carefully to see if there is any particular cause. Sometimes the doctor will have to refer the person to hospital.

STROKE

If you have had one stroke this does not necessarily mean you will have a second, and there are steps that can be taken to reduce the risk of a second stroke. Go to see your doctor and ask if there are ways in which you could reduce your risk of a second stroke. Ask the doctor if he or she thinks that aspirin taken regularly would help.

Common Health Problems

There are a number of health problems, as distinct from diseases, which occur in old age. (Diseases can be diagnosed only by a doctor, but health problems can be identified by everybody.) These problems may come on slowly, and can sometimes (though not always) be the first signs of disease in old age. For this reason you should always see a doctor if you develop one or more of the following common health problems: breathlessness; incontinence; difficulty in getting a good night's sleep; stiffness; tiredness and weakness; pain.

Breathlessness
Most people get breathless more easily at seventy than at twenty, but you should see your doctor if:

- Breathlessness limits your ability to carry out any essential tasks such as climbing a flight of stairs.
- You notice you are breathless when you are sitting still or you wake up at night breathless.
- Breathlessness is accompanied by chest pain.
- You notice that you are getting breathless more quickly.

Your doctor will examine you, paying particular attention to your lungs, heart and blood pressure. He may send off a blood sample for testing or request a chest X-ray or ECG (a test which examines the way in which your heart is working). If no disease is found, the doctor may give you advice about increasing the amount of exercise you take to get fitter, because breathlessness is a sign of unfitness as well as a sign of disease. If a disease is found, the doctor may start treatment.

If the doctor is puzzled by your case or finds the disease difficult to manage, he can refer you to a consultant physician; or, if the disease results from heart problems, to a cardiologist; or, if your breathlessness comes from lung problems, such as bronchitis or emphysema, to a consultant in chest medicine.

Sometimes people do not realize that they are becoming more breathless and you may notice it, for example, in a friend whom you have not seen for a long time.

Urinary Incontinence in Men

When a group of retired men gather together, it is uncommon for that group not to know at least one man who has had 'troublesome waterworks'.

At the lower end of the bladder in men lies the prostate gland. This swells with age, probably as the result of normal ageing, and in some men it swells more than in others, for no known reason, obstructing the passage of urine from the bladder to the outside. The first symptoms are difficulties in starting to pass water and dribbling at the end of the stream. Sometimes, however, the first warning of prostate trouble is that the man develops what is called an acute retention of urine in which he is completely unable to pass water, but this usually occurs because the man has had to go to bed for some other reason – for example, after an operation or as the result of a heart attack.

As soon as a man notices difficulty with passing water he should consult his doctor who may refer him to a consultant surgeon to see whether a prostate operation is needed.

Urinary Incontinence and Other Urinary Problems in Women

Because of their anatomical differences, women experience very different urinary problems from those suffered by men. Women have two common urinary problems – incontinence (or dribbling) and infections.

Very many women have difficulty holding their water. The usual cause is that the muscles of the floor of the pelvis, on which the bladder sits and through which urine passes, have been weakened and stretched by childbirth. The first symptoms may be the passing of small amounts of urine when the woman coughs, laughs or strains – for example, when trying to push something heavy or lifting a child. The best approach to this type of problem is to try to strengthen the muscles in the pelvic floor by exercising them. This can be done by stopping the flow of urine in mid-stream and holding it for a short time (count to 10), then letting go and repeating the exercise. This should be done every time you go to the toilet. Another way to strengthen the pelvic floor muscles is to imagine that you are in a lift and going up several floors as you tighten your bladder muscles to their limit before releasing them slowly again as the lift goes down.

Another common urinary problem among women is cystitis, the symptoms of which are discomfort in passing urine, the frequent feeling that they should pass urine, and urgency or very great desire to pass urine at short notice even though there may not be very much urine in the bladder. Sometimes cystitis is caused by bacteria which can be treated, but on other occasions it is not possible for the doctor to find any cause that can be treated with antibiotics. One approach is for the sufferer to drink lots of water but the topic of cystitis is a complex one and women who experience the problem are advised to read a book about it, such as *Understanding Cystitis* by Angela Kilmartin (published by Arrow).

Soiling and Problems with the Back Passage

The most common cause of soiling, or the passage of small amounts of faeces which make underpants or bedclothes soiled, is constipation: chronic constipation causes the bowel to secrete more mucus than usual and this can leak out. The best way to prevent this problem is to increase the amount of fibre in the diet – with caution. Large amounts of fibre consumed by people who are not used to it can have results that are literally explosive and may result in one or more real episodes of incontinence of faeces. Start with wholemeal bread and fruit before moving on to pure bran or high-fibre breakfast cereals. Dietary fibre is discussed in more detail in the *Saga Food Guide*, also in this series.

In most other cases incontinence is secondary to some other more serious disease, such as a stroke, and the person affected will be receiving help on account of that disease.

Difficulty in Getting a Good Night's Sleep

A good night's sleep is important for two reasons: first, sleep is necessary for good health; and second, failure to sleep is itself a common cause of anxiety and can set up a cycle in which the person tries so hard to go to sleep that he or she is even less successful at doing so.

Different people have different ideas about what is a good night's sleep. Margaret Thatcher, for example, is said never to need more than six hours' sleep and Napoleon claimed that more than five hours was an unnecessary luxury, but many people need eight or

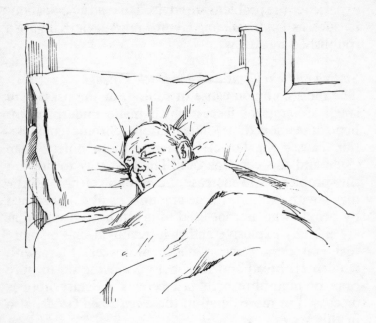

nine hours to function effectively. Most people probably need about seven hours' sleep to function well.

The common causes of sleep problems are:

- Physical illnesses which cause pain, discomfort or distressing symptoms that can keep you awake or rouse you in the middle of the night. If you find that your sleep is disturbed by pain or by symptoms such as breathlessness or the need to pass water, see your doctor.
- Anxiety. If you cannot get to sleep at night because some problem is on your mind, you need to tackle that problem. Seek an appropriate source of help and find someone you like, trust and respect to give you support during the time that the cause of the anxiety is being dealt with.

- Depression. This can be a cause of early-morning waking. Even if you cannot identify any obvious cause of your depression, or just feel generally run down rather than being depressed about any particular thing, see your doctor.
- Daytime napping. There is nothing wrong with taking a nap after lunch, but it is unrealistic to expect that you will sleep equally well at night if you do.
- A disorganized evening. This is a common cause of disturbed sleep and is discussed in more detail below.

SETTING A REGULAR BEDTIME PATTERN

A number of people develop sleep problems because they have a disorganized evening. In some cases this is because, in seeking to overcome another sleep problem, they try all manner of different techniques, often a new one each evening, in an attempt to find the 'cure', thus destroying any routine and making things worse. This is not the way to tackle difficulty with sleeping. The most important step to take is to establish a regular pattern of bedtime activities – for example, by ensuring that you have the following:

- No television after 10.30pm and no exciting or violent television after 9.30pm.
- Something soothing to read and a warm drink before going upstairs.
- A warm bath.
- A warm bed into which you climb at almost the same time every night.
- Something gentle to read or listen to before going to sleep.
- Lights out at about the same time every night.

If you have difficulty in sleeping, try this for a month and see what happens.

ARE SLEEPING TABLETS EFFECTIVE?
The answer is that they are effective: sleeping tablets do help you sleep. Unfortunately, however, they have side effects such as sleepiness the next morning. Even more serious is the fact that some people can become dependent on them, and when they are unable to sleep without them have to spend the rest of their life taking sleeping tablets, sometimes in increasing doses.

If you ask your doctor for sleeping tablets, or if he or she suggests them, remember that it is important to take them for only one month, in part as a trial, in part to get you back into regular sleeping, and then to return to depending on the natural daily rhythm of the body which produces sleep once every twenty-four hours if you help it by a regular evening ritual.

Stiffness
Everybody gets a little stiffer as they get older. If, however, you find stiffness affecting your ability to dress in the morning or perform any of the common household tasks such as having a bath, doing housework or undressing at night, you should seek help.

Stiffness is almost always due to a form of arthritis, and this often requires medical treatment, but you can do a great deal to help yourself. The most important thing is to keep active and supple, and the range of suppleness exercises described on page 39 will be useful to you if you have arthritis. In addition swimming is excellent, because the water lessens the weight of your body and allows your joints to work more easily. Do not exercise your joints if they are painful, though; and do not force your joints to move into any position that is not natural to them, but strive to maintain and improve your suppleness and strength, within your own limits.

Foot Problems

Painful feet are a specially unpleasant aspect of arthritis because they can limit the distance you are able to walk. Other problems occur on the skin of the feet, but almost all of the foot problems older people experience result from arthritis either because this disease affects the bones and joints of the feet or because its presence elsewhere in the body makes it difficult for them to look after their feet properly. People who have diabetes or narrowing of the arteries in the legs are particularly prone to develop ulcers on their feet.

Care of the feet includes regular washing and careful drying and great caution in cutting toenails: cut them straight across and do not round the corners as this can lead to ingrowing toenails. In addition try to buy and wear comfortable shoes; you may also find pads under the ball of your foot helpful in relieving pain.

However, it is often wise to consult a chiropodist regarding any foot problems you may have. The NHS runs a chiropody service, but this is frequently under great pressure, and although you should always try for NHS chiropody (ask your GP how you can obtain it), you may have to go for private treatment. If you do, always choose someone who is a state registered chiropodist.

Pain

Pain is not a normal consequence of ageing.

Chest pain should always be taken seriously; and if

you develop pain in the chest which may go up into the neck or the left arm, you should phone your doctor immediately. Often such pain is not followed by a heart attack, but it is better to be safe than sorry.

Obviously, any very severe pain should be treated as an emergency, but most of the pain that occurs is not a medical emergency. Sometimes pain will go away as quickly as it came, but you should see your doctor about persistent pain. If you have pain for days and months on end, you have a tremendous problem to bear. Pain killers by themselves can be effective, but severe pain may be difficult to control with ordinary pain killers. There are pain clinics in the NHS which can help people with severe pain, but some people find acupuncture or other forms of treatment helpful. Chiropractors and osteopaths can help people with longstanding back or neck pain.

Common Disabilities

Disability is not the result of normal ageing until very advanced old age. If you reach the age of ninety and have kept yourself reasonably fit and active, you should be able to:

- Dress and undress.
- Get to the toilet in time.
- Have a bath or wash all over.
- Do housework and gardening – at least the light jobs, if not the heavy ones.
- Shop for and prepare the food you want to eat.

If you lose the ability to perform any of these tasks, you should not assume that it is the result of 'old age', and you should not accept it if someone else asks you,

'What else can you expect at your age?' It is important to remember that the onset of disease in old age may be indicated by changes not commonly considered to be symptoms of disease, as in the following example.

John S retired fit and well at sixty-three, and in the first few years of his retirement played more golf than he had done during the last few years of his working life when he was particularly busy. His handicap was 12 and he actually improved this in the year after retirement. At the age of sixty-seven, however, he found that he could no longer play a full round of golf, partly because he was feeling tired at about the ninth hole, and partly because he found the steep hill up the fifteenth green getting too much for him; he had to stop for breath half-way up it. Because he found eighteen holes too much, he stopped playing with the friends with whom he had formerly played, and took to playing only an easy loop of seven holes by himself.

John S may have had no option but to give up playing eighteen holes but he should certainly have consulted his doctor, because it is not normal ageing to become unable to play eighteen holes of golf suddenly at the age of sixty-seven; something else was going on which should have been investigated.

Helping Someone with Disabilities

Even the professionals now recognize that most care is provided not by highly trained and highly paid professionals but by disabled people themselves, providing self-care, and relative and neighbours. When Health Service employees talk about 'elderly people' or patients in a department of geriatric medicine, they are not thinking of sixty- and seventy-year-olds but of people in their late eighties and nineties, and anyone who works in the Health Service with these very elderly patients soon learns that much of the care is provided either by a husband or wife, themselves in their late eighties or nineties, or by relatives, many of whom are in their fifties and sixties.

Each disabled person has his or her own pattern of disabilities which presents particular challenges to caring relatives, but there are a small number of general principles which the carers themselves should bear in mind:

1 Think of your own health first. Too often people who are looking after disabled relatives suffer unnecessary health problems themselves for one or more of the following reasons:

(a) They do not recognize that they are developing an illness because they assume that they are simply tired when they are in fact ill.

(b) They are thinking so much about the disabled older person that they do not think about their own health.

(c) The stress of caring can in itself make people more susceptible to disease.

(d) All the attention of the family and the professionals involved may focus on the disabled person, thus leading to the carer's health problems being overlooked.

If you are looking after somebody and are feeling unwell, the best plan is not just to mention this fact to the doctor when he or she comes to visit the disabled person, but to make an appointment of your own and find some time when you can speak to the doctor solely about your problem. Think of your own health and take steps to improve it. This is not selfish, for ultimately it will be to the benefit of the disabled person in your charge: you will not be able to care for him or her if your own health breaks down.

2 Always look for ways in which the health of the disabled person could be improved. It is all too easy, when looking after somebody who is very disabled, to assume that all their problems are due to the combined effects of advanced old age and disease and that nothing can be done to alleviate these. But disabled people may develop acute health problems or they may suffer a relapse in their condition which could be dealt with by good medical care. It is sometimes therefore worth asking if a second opinion could be obtained and it is usually possible to do this without offending your own GP's feelings by suggesting that you would like the person in your care to have some physiotherapy to see if this would improve their level of ability. GPs cannot usually arrange physiotherapy themselves but have to refer patients to a hospital department for physiotherapy. This usually results in their medical condition being reviewed as well as the need for physiotherapy.

If the problems have suddenly become worse because of a deterioration in the disabled person's ability, or simply if you feel desperate, consider asking for a hospital referral either to the department of geriatric medicine or, if the problem is Alzheimer's disease (senile dementia), to a psychiatric hospital department specializing in the problems of elderly people with mental infirmity.

3 See what steps can be taken to solve practical problems such as those concerning housing or low

income. If, for example, you are a single daughter looking after an elderly parent or parents, you need to be sure that your housing is secure after the death of your parents. *The Saga Property Guide* and *The Saga Money Guide*, also in this series, will provide you with useful information, and should help you solve practical problems.

4 Find substitutes for the help you are giving. It is sometimes possible to provide substitute care for that which you are providing. For example, to relieve caring relatives from having to travel every day to make a meal, the meals on wheels service may be provided to people who cannot prepare their own food. Similarly, the home help service is available to relieve a relative who is getting worn down or suffering stress as a result of the need to provide daily home care. This is now recognized by home help services as a good reason for providing help for old people in their own homes. Likewise, the district nursing service (see page 67) may be able to provide help to bathe someone to relieve a relative either of the physical strain or the embarrassment of bathing their parent.

Obviously the home help organizers are grateful for any help that a relative can give and when the pressure on them is great, as it almost always is, try to give most help to those elderly and disabled people who have no relatives. However, most organizers are now usually sympathetic to the problems of caring relatives and do not refuse to provide help for older people simply because they believe that a son or daughter 'should' provide all the care required.

5 Getting regular relief. There are two main ways in which relief can be provided:

(a) The disabled elderly person may attend a day centre or day hospital so that on one or more days a week the caring relative is freed from the burden of looking after and the anxiety of worrying about the old person on their own. Ask a doctor, district nurse or health visitor about day hospital and day care facilities in the area in which the disabled older person lives. In general, day hospitals provide care for only ten or twelve weeks, during which time they try to help the older person get fitter, but they do sometimes provide long-term care for those older people who are too disabled for social services day centres to look after. To get a place at a local authority day centre you will have to approach the local Social Services Department.

(b) Another very effective way of providing relief for carers is to offer the disabled person regular admissions to an old people's home or hospital. These admissions may be every weekend, or one week in four, or one week in six, or some combination which helps both the old person and his or her carer. The disabled person may be reluctant to go at first, and it may take the advice of an outsider for him or her to appreciate that the reason he or she is being asked to go to a hospital or old people's home regularly is not that the carer no longer loves him or her, but that the carer has to have this relief to allow him or her to continue the care.

Further Information
Caring for Older People – A Practical Guide for Everyone, by J.A. Muir Gray and Heather Mackenzie, published by Penguin in 1986, covers in more detail the topics touched on above.

In addition the National Council for Carers and their Elderly Dependants, 29 Chilworth Mews, London W2 3RG (tel: 01–262 1451) can also advise on this type of problem. Locally Age Concern or the Community Health Council can advise on the services that are available and how those services can be mobilized to help carers continue caring.

USEFUL ADDRESSES

Alzheimer's Disease Society
40 Shandwick Place
Edinburgh
Scotland
Tel: 031-225 1453

Chest, Heart and Stroke Association
Tavistock House
Tavistock Square
London WC1H 9JE
Tel: 01-387 3012

Citizens Advice Bureau
Look in your local phone book for the address of your
nearest office. Helps with information on benefits and
services in your area.

Counsel and Care for the Elderly
131 Middlesex Street
London E1
Tel: 01-621 1624

Disabled Living Foundation
380-384 Harrow Road
London W9 2HU
Tel: 01-289 6111

MIND (National Association for Mental Health)
22 Harley Street
London W1N 2ED
Tel: 01-637 0741

National Council for Carers and their Elderly
Dependants (NCCED)
29 Chilworth Mews
London W2 3RG
Tel: 01-262 1451

National Society for Cancer Relief
Michael Sobell House
30 Dorset Square
London NW1 6OL
Tel: 01-402 8125

Parkinson's Disease Society
36 Portland Place
London W1N 3DG
Tel: 01-323 1174

Royal National Institute for the Deaf
105 Gower Street
London WC1 6AH
Tel: 01-387 8033

Royal National Institute for the Blind
224 Great Portland Street
London W1N 6AA
Tel: 01-388 1266

saga
RIGHTS GUIDE

This guide clearly outlines the many rights, concessions and services which become available to you on your retirement.

- Pensions, both within the UK and abroad
- Illness and disability provisions
- Help with a low income • Rate and rent rebates
- Legal aid • Motor insurance

These are just some of the issues clarified in this book. Concluding with useful addresses, and information about complaints procedures and ombudsmen, this is an essential reference book to steer you through today's complex bureaucracy.

Paul Lewis is a freelance writer who contributes regularly to *Saga Magazine*, and is an expert on financial and legal matters.

Other books in this series

Saga Property Guide
Saga Food Guide
Saga Money Guide
Saga Leisure Guide

saga

PROPERTY GUIDE

Retirement is a time when many of us reassess our housing requirements, and start to look to the future. This book gives practical common sense advice on all the concerns that most often arise, including:

- The pros and cons of moving to a smaller home
- Holiday resorts • Sheltered Housing
- Living abroad • Nursing homes
- Buying and selling property
- Legal and financial aspects

Concluding with lists of addresses of builders, trade and aid organizations specializing in retirement housing, this invaluable guide will equip you to take the housing decisions best suited to your needs.

Michael Dineen is a regular Saga contributor and writes a weekly property column for *The Observer*.

Other books in this series

Saga Rights Guide
Saga Money Guide
Saga Leisure Guide
Saga Food Guide

saga
MONEY GUIDE

For all of us, retirement brings a change in our financial position. This clear, practical guide will help you plan and manage your money in the best possible way for a secure and happy retirement. It includes advice on:

- Company and private pensions
- Income and inheritance tax
- Investing in the Stock Market • Gifts
- Insurance • Making a will

Complete with useful addresses and information on how to get specialist advice, this easy-to-follow book will allow you to get the best possible financial deal for your long term future.

Paul Lewis is a freelance writer who contributes regularly to *Saga Magazine*, and is an expert on financial and legal matters.

Other books in this series

Saga Property Guide
Saga Health Guide
Saga Leisure Guide
Saga Rights Guide

saga
LEISURE GUIDE

Your retirement is the opportunity to do all those things
you've hoped to do but never had the time.

- Long distance luxury cruises
- Weekend breaks • Caravanning
- University courses • Charity work
- New sports and pastimes

These are just some of the many ideas explored in this book.
The *Saga Leisure Guide* includes a questionnaire on your
qualities as a retiree and offers advice on courses to prepare
you for this new phase. This is the book to ensure that your
retirement is the time of your life.

Roy Johnstone is a freelance journalist and a regular
contributor to *Saga Magazine* on leisure issues.

Other books in this series

Saga Property Guide
Saga Food Guide
Saga Money Guide
Saga Rights Guide

saga
FOOD GUIDE

Retirement is an excellent time to take more pleasure in cooking and enjoying your food – and a time to improve your diet to keep in good shape. This book is full of advice and inspiration on subjects such as:

- Basic nutrition ● Cooking for one or two
- Tips for beginners ● Entertaining
- Good value meals ● Convenience foods
- Catering for grandchildren ● Picnics
- Clever shopping

Each section ends with two or three recipes, and the book includes advice on specialist diets, vegetarianism, fats and fibres.

Carol Leverkus is a freelance nutritionist with a special interest in healthy diets for the retirement age group.

Other books in this series

Saga Rights Guide
Saga Money Guide
Saga Leisure Guide
Saga Property Guide